# Inner Gifts Uncovered

# Inner Gifts Uncovered
## The Complete Reiki 2nd Degree Manual

Continuing on the Path of
Self Empowerment and Reiki

Marnie Vincolisi

This book is not intended as a substitute for the medical recommendations of physicians or other health-care providers. Rather, it is intended to offer alternative information to help the reader cooperate with physicians and health professionals in a mutual quest for optimal well-being and a better understanding of self.

Published by Light Internal
Littleton, Colorado
www.lightinternal.com

Cover design by Rich Allen
Photograph of author by Robert Leichtenberg

ISBN     978-0-9823732-1-7                    Price   $13.95

*Dedication*

This book is dedicated to every soul
who searches for the power within.

*Be yourself. No one can ever tell you you're doing it wrong.*

James Leo Herlihy

*May your life journey be one of discovery, joy, compassion and love, and may all these qualities be claimed by you.*

*Marnie Vincolisi*

# Table of Contents

*Chapter 5*

*Chapter 6*

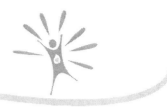

# Introduction

Reiki holds the story of a man who spent a good portion of his life searching for truth as he followed his passion of healing. In his service to others he was blessed. His quest took him not only traveling to physical places but deep within his soul as well, for no gift can be given to another until it is found within ones' own being. This book and the teachings found in the second degree of Reiki have the ability to uncover the truth which lies within you.

Healing or curiosity may be the first reason you searched for Reiki, but as you continue on your journey through the levels of Reiki you will find it takes you along a path which will have turns you never expected. There are treasures inside of you which have only been slightly revealed with the attunement of first degree Reiki. The opening which occurs is often profound, yet it is only the beginning of a tour through the inherent gifts which are yours and yours alone.

Only you can find your gifts, no one else has the key to open these doors and the surprise will be ruined if you entrust another to reveal these accolades to you. When you turn to a master for assistance, know they are only guides. They can direct, but the power comes from discovering the information for yourself. The visions held by others are from their perspective and from their sight it can be askew. When seen through your own eyes the vision is clearly your message unclouded by the concepts of another. This then becomes your truth, one which cannot be denied.

I have seen it happen many times: a student will appear curious about the attributes held within Reiki and once they are attuned to Reiki the changes begin. New ideas are presented to them through books, movies, conversations or in the press. This information has been dormant within their field of consciousness and then as their awareness widens the change becomes more prevalent. As one door is opened, other doorways of opportunity soon appear. As the first year passes, the initiate is walking and talking in ways that were foreign in the past. Thoughts have power and the student soon discovers what can be done while simply directing their mind onto a positive path. New opportunities arise in places unexpected. Old patterns fall away as new people appear in order to support this new way of life.

One may surmise change is a natural progression through life and growth inevitably happens, but is this completely true? From what I have observed I venture to say nay. I see so many souls searching for a better job, a loving partner, a relationship with a parent, a purpose in life, but the underlying desire is not simply in finding these connections, but rather in discovering love. And that love will only start when it is found within our own hearts; this is what Reiki reveals.

If you look within your circle of acquaintances, do you notice that people, who search for love outside of themselves, do not move forward into their dreams unless they make a major change in their life? That change is acceptance. Of what was and what will be. To make this leap they require support and guidance and they do not always find it. For within each of these desires holds emptiness, a hole which can only be filled when one knows there is *nothing outside of us which cannot be found within us.*

All my life I looked for love. My parents were divorced before I was born, which left a hole in my heart. Because of misunderstandings between my mother and father and their families, my father and I were not allowed to meet. My search for love seemed to end when I was 40 years old and I first met my dad and his family. I was living in Denver and he in Chicago. When we finally met I thought, "This is the love I have been looking for all my life!" My heart was full. But unfortunately, three months after I met my dad, he passed from his body with lung cancer, which could have left my heart empty again. The love carrot, which dangled out in front of me all my life, was given and then quickly taken away.

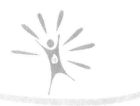

When I found my dad I discovered his illness was terminal and because of that I treasured every conversation we had, brief as they were. I was hoping his love would fill the emptiness in my heart but, alas, it did not. He had difficulty speaking and it took him a long time to present his thoughts and form the words. As he slowly formed a sentence he would lose his train of thought and the reason to converse was lost and I never heard what he was trying to tell me. This became frustrating for not only me, but him as well. All those years were gone and now his heart desires of the past could not be expressed.

Gifts in life are held in moments, not words. I could have let my disappointment and desire to hear his loving thoughts consume me but it would not have served either one of us. I was able to find the moment which showed me his love, far beyond what words could express. It was just a flash in time but it is embedded in my memory for life. Only an hour after I knocked on the door of my dad's home I was in his car going to see his sisters. He was so delighted I found him that he wanted to share his joy with his family immediately. One week prior, one of his three sisters had passed on so many of my cousins from around the country were at my uncle's home that Sunday afternoon.

We exited his car on the way to the house and I began to walk along the sidewalk next to my dad. He, just as naturally as breathing, reached down and held my hand. We walked a short distance to Uncle Mario's home, hand in hand and I thought to myself, "Life does not get any better than this. Here I am, walking with my dad and he is holding my hand." In that moment I felt the 40 years of his love, all that he would have bestowed upon me if he had the chance. What a precious moment.

My life as a child and with my family was not the ideal scenario I had in mind for my life. I did not want to be the outcast and yet I felt I was. It was the 1950's and I really was the only girl in school without a father and yet it seemed okay... it was all I knew. Somehow, it was all perfect. For there is no model family, no "right" job, no divine partner, no ultimate purpose. Love is all there is and it is ultimately found inside you. My father, in his absence, gave me a gift so I would have to locate my own heart's love, for without him around I had to search for love in my own heart. He showed me his love briefly and then left, leaving his mark of compassion. Through this experience, the door to my heart was opened but it still took years to fill the void and find my intimate partner. I took time during this interlude to find love within my own heart. I waited for true love to find me but it did take longer than I had anticipated. For there is no timeline for love; it happens when all the stars are in alignment and certain experiences have been met by both individuals. There is no rushing it.

The beauty of Reiki is the gift it channels, which is pure love. In this space during a treatment or an attunement, time falls away and life can be enjoyed in the moment. One cannot be touched by this loving energy without opening one's heart. It would be virtually impossible because Reiki flows through the head, heart and hands, thus creating this access. It's through this window that the heart is filled with compassion and the experiences of life are perceived in a new softer light.

I have encountered some who say they do not feel the power of Reiki, that it does not work for them. Yet after they are introduced to Reiki either by a treatment or a class, I see their life beginning to change. The differences can be profound and obvious or subtle as a sleeping giant. I have said it once and I will say it again and again: Reiki works 100% of the time. It will quietly make its mark within one or any of the four bodies: physical, mental, emotional or spiritual. To an untrained eye these changes may go unnoticed, hence the observation that nothing is happening. But to the one who can see within, the changes are tremendous. Second degree Reiki will reveal this gift of inner sight to you. Use it wisely. It is not given to make judgments of what is intuitively seen; it is given to draw out compassion for self and others.

My path with Reiki began when I was energetically pushed out of my old vocation, presenting a need to develop a new business, free from the stress of the past. I had no idea where to start. I dissolved my previous toy business before I

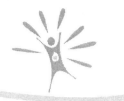

knew the next step to take. My path appeared to be out of order; certainly I should know how I am going to make a living before I disband my company. But life does not always present opportunities in the order we feel we require, yet it is always in divine order. I was being taught to trust the process and from my acceptance of what was to be, my next step appeared.

The second degree of Reiki training will push you into the next phase of your life path. There is no turning around. As in the movie *Matrix* Neo had a choice to take one of two pills. He was cautioned once he took the red pill there was no turning back. It is true! Once you step onto the path of consciousness you will not be able to close your eyes to the underlying truth around you. Once awakened, reality and truth will not go unseen ever again.

There are processes in this book called "Life Tools," to assist in this venture. They will allow you to peer through the looking glass into your own psyche and, with love, move you to the other side. Any of these processes cannot be done incorrectly. If the intent is to assist yourself or another, the request shall be granted. When Reiki is added to the mix, love flows and all is placed in divine order. So do not fret, you do not have to follow this manual as it is exactly stated. Allow your intuition to direct you; this book carries a guideline, that is all.

Revisit this publication from time to time, as you will find new discoveries each time. When you are troubled you may find as you thumb through the book the answer will appear to be revealed. Trust your own intuition. You will find it to be your best guide.

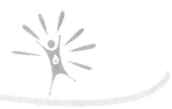

# Chapter 1

## Understanding the History

Mikao Usui was a minister that lived in Kyoto, Japan, whose life made a turn when one of his students at Doshisha University asked, "Do you accept the contents of the Bible literally?" Usui answered that he did. The student continued his questions.

"You believe Jesus walked upon the water and healed the sick even though you have not seen this happen?" Usui again agreed that he did.

The student probed even more. "This is enough for you to believe on blind faith. You have lived your life and are secure. I am young, just starting on my path, I need more proof."

The questions asked of Usui began to plague his mind. He began to wonder how indeed Jesus did perform such healing miracles. His mind would not be still so Usui left his position as president of Doshisha University and came to the United

States to search for the truth of how Jesus healed. Surely the answers must be within the written documents treasured in the Christian religions of the world. Much to his dismay, when he received his doctorate degree in scripture at the University of Chicago, he still had not attained the knowledge which would give him the ability to aid the ill and alleviate pain. He sadly returned to his home land of Japan.

Perhaps it was time to look within the religious philosophies of his own country. Usui had heard that Buddha had the ability to make the body whole, so he continued his study of healing at various Buddhist monasteries. When questioned about the healing attributes of Buddha, the monks told him they no longer possessed the ability to heal as Buddha did, for their focus was now on the healing of the soul.

So Usui continued his search which led him to manuscripts written in Chinese and Sanskrit. He learned to translate a wider range of writings, but still had no success in his quest to find how to apply healing to others. At last, within ancient Sanskrit text, he found what he was looking for: the knowledge and symbols on how to heal the body. But his efforts were in vain, for he still did not obtain the ability to perform the healing himself. Usui shared his concerns with a Zen monk, who suggested that he meditate for 21 days on the holy mountain of Mount Kuri Yama, as many monks had done before him. His meditation was to be focused upon the ability to heal.

For days he sat alone on the mountain, contemplating, praying and observing subtle energy shifts. On the last day on the mountain, Usui had a spiritual experience he was waiting for. A beam of light from a distant star hit him in his third eye and knocked him out cold.

In his unconscious state, he envisioned bubbles of light containing the symbols he had discovered in the ancient Sanskrit sutras. Upon awakening, he was unclear as to what had happened, but he soon discovered that he had attained what he

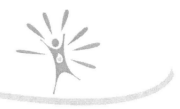

was seeking: the ability to heal. From that point on, Usui dedicated his life to healing the sick. He practiced for many years in the beggars' quarters of Japan.

Although the traditional story passed down over 100 years about the originator of Reiki is well accepted in the healing community, there are parts of this story that never totally resonated with me. In my heart, I did not believe Usui was a Christian minister or that he journeyed to America. Even the symbols he found in the Sanskrit sutras did not feel correct to me. My suspicions were confirmed when I found and read *Reiki Fire* by Frank Petter. Petter traveled to Japan and uncovered what he felt was the truth about Usui. He found that Usui was a businessman who was interested in healing and that Usui did venture up Mount Kuri Yama to search for his healing ability. Petter also discovered that Usui was never a minister, he was not a monk, and he did not work in the beggars' quarters. To add to the mystery, there is no record in the University of Chicago showing the enrollment of Usui.

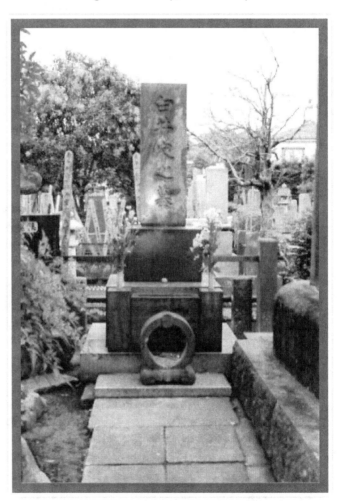

Usui family gravestone

Some say Usui never even existed, yet Petter found Usui's family gravestone and reports how to locate this stone in his book. If you venture to Japan, perhaps you would like to do a bit of research yourself. But let us consider, does it matter if he lived or not?

What is important is the change Reiki has made in so many lives. And how it can be felt and channeled as it assists others to grow and heal deep within their spirit. So why all the mystery?

If we start by looking at the lineage of Reiki we can begin to understand where the misconceptions began. Mikao Usui is the originator of Reiki, he trained about a dozen masters and appointed Chujiro Hayashi to be the next Grand Master. Hayashi in turn also trained many masters; all but one were male and he selected the only female he trained, Hawayo Takata, to be the Grand Master to follow him. The title of Grand Master no longer exists either in the Usui traditional lineage or in non-traditional Reiki. As we learn and apply our healing gifts, we can all be our own Grand Masters. I tell my students there is no need to call me Grand Master for I prefer Goddess.

The concept of Gurus and masters is an old paradigm concept. In the past, initiates of various studies felt the only way to enlightenment was to blindly follow a dogma or masters who have already walked the path they were seeking. Times have changed; the vibration of the earth is raised by those who have gone before us. Now we have stepped into a time where we can claim our personal connection to the higher intelligence which encompasses us without giving away our power to another by seeing them above us. We all have the same opportunity to advance using our inherent abilities. A real master will guide the initiate to uncover their gifts, thus revealing their own brilliance.

Each Grand Master had their special gifts; Hayashi was not only a doctor but also a proficient master of martial arts. He observed that as the ancient practices were taken out of the country of Japan, they changed. Hayashi felt this was a dishonoring of the practice. Takata was Japanese but had moved to Hawaii.

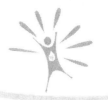

Because of ill health she returned to Japan to seek healing. She was a client in Hayashi's clinic and became interested in Reiki because of the profound healing she had received. It took much coaching by Takata to convince Hayashi to teach her Reiki. His concern was that if he taught Hawayo Takata and named her the next Grand Master, she may leave the county with the knowledge and perhaps Reiki would not be honored by foreigners and the practice would be changed. He did not understand that we all have divine gifts which when added to the Reiki discipline will enhance it and empower the user as well as the recipient.

Hayashi instructed Takata to stay in Japan until the war ended, for he also knew that, as a Japanese American, she would be in danger if she returned to Hawaii. Takata became the director of Hayashi's clinic in Japan and practiced there for years after he passed from his body. When she finally returned to Hawaii around 1950, she felt Americans might not readily accept a Japanese healing modality because of the effects of the war and Pearl Harbor. It is my understanding she created the Christian story about Usui so that Reiki would be more palatable to American students. Hence, the mystery begins to unfold.

Another misconception is how Usui received the sacred Reiki symbols. The symbols were understood to be from Tibetan Sanskrit sutras, but we observe that they are written in Japanese. The question arises: if Usui found the symbols in Tibetan writings, then why are they now written in another language? If Usui discovered the symbols in the Sanskrit writings, then why are they not written in Sanskrit? Could Usui's guides have translated the symbols which rained down upon him during his spiritual awakening upon the mountain?

Just as Americans may not have readily accepted esoteric instruction from a Japanese foreigner, the people of Japan perhaps would have difficulty accepting the symbols if they were presented in Sanskrit. Within the divine knowledge of Usui's guides, the adjustments may have been made and the symbols translated into Japanese.

The symbols we see today have also been adjusted for the American culture as a gift from our Reiki guides. The distant symbol is rather lengthy, creating a challenge in itself to memorize. If the symbol also had to be drawn from bottom to top and right to left as they write in the Orient, its difficulty would be greatly increased. The adjustment has been made for our symbols to be written according to our western style, thus increasing our ability to draw and remember them.

The history of Reiki has been handed down by word of mouth. No one really knows the truth, hence the enigma. In the non-traditional approach to Reiki, the trick is to find the account which resonates within you and then release your attachment to this story. It does not matter what accuracy the fable holds; the power of Reiki lies within each individual. The attunement process awakens a natural ability to heal and immediately raises the vibration of the body so the power can be accessed and used. The change is automatic; the initiate need not do a thing to receive the gift during the transfer process. It flows in and the result is instantly embraced. Therefore its origin is unimportant.

Usui experienced many of the challenges we have today. His business at one point had failed, but this did not deter him from searching for his spiritual path. He went on not only to find his healing gifts, but also helping others to reach their transcendence. His teachings have stood the test of time. Today, many students are realizing they can experience life changing energy with just a little practice. Reiki represents a path to greater fulfillment and success, in life and in spirit. Though Reiki might appear to only be for healing, it moves far beyond its simple sustaining health benefits. As you move into your next level of Reiki this truth will become more apparent.

Another fallacy is held in the Original Principles of Reiki, for they were not written by Usui, but adopted by him from the Meiji Emperor of Japan. The Emperor, who lived from 1868 to 1912, set down these principles for the people of his country as guidance for a fulfilled life. There are various translations which all support the basic Christian golden rule, "Do unto others as you would have them do unto you."

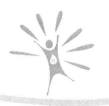

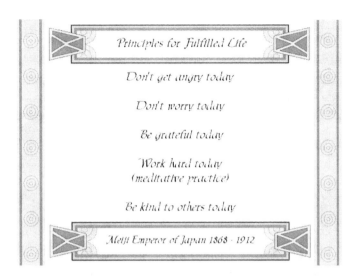

> Principles for Fulfilled Life
>
> *Don't get angry today*
>
> *Don't worry today*
>
> *Be grateful today*
>
> *Work hard today*
> *(meditative practice)*
>
> *Be kind to others today*
>
> Meiji Emperor of Japan 1868 - 1912

Every time you move up a level in Reiki, on some level you agree to abide by some or all of these principles. And as you do your abilities increase as your heart expands.

Notice the similarities between The Principles for a Fulfilled Life, from the Emperor and The Principles of Reiki, from Usui. They address worry, anger, gratitude, kindness, practice and love. These principles reflect attributes that would be desired and honored by anyone who was looking to produce harmony in their life. Reiki is not a practice which is given intermittently; it is a life style choice as referenced in the principles. To walk the path of Reiki is to live it every day.

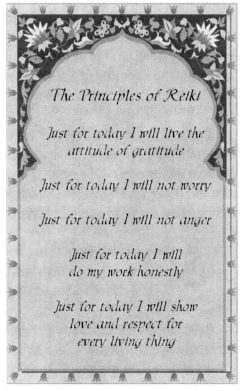

> The Principles of Reiki
>
> *Just for today I will live the attitude of gratitude*
>
> *Just for today I will not worry*
>
> *Just for today I will not anger*
>
> *Just for today I will do my work honestly*
>
> *Just for today I will show love and respect for every living thing*

It is through the focused practice of compassion wherein the gift of Reiki expands. This *benevolence* needs to be bestowed upon the self before it can be truly felt and accepted when given to another. Reiki begins to illumine and open an honesty which was previously denied. When an old situation is seen in a new light, the healing deepens. The radiance of Reiki is what gives this process ease and grace.

## Second Degree Reiki

The decision to advance to Second Degree Reiki is a step up onto the rungs of the ladder which leads one into yet another growth pattern. With this attunement, the crown and third eye chakra will become increasingly clearer and the results will be reflected with accelerated intuition. These attunements will square the Reiki energy of the level one initiate, opening up even more healing energies. The squaring of the energy is more than doubled. It is the energy times itself which transmutes an enormous change.

There will also be increased sensitivity in the hands for those chakras were only partially opened in the first degree Reiki attunement and now the hand chakras will become fully open. This will give the practitioner the ability to plug into the chakra system of the recipient, thus allowing for a clearer reading of information in the recipient's body and psyche.

 **Remember:** Even though the practitioner will be more connected to the client, the practitioner will not transfer the client's issues into their own body.

Reiki is a process of channeling energy. This creates a light barrier so the client's issues and aliments are self contained and allowed to release into the ethers rather than the practitioner's body.

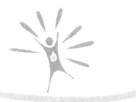

Every time a student moves up to a higher degree of Reiki, the communication with their spiritual guides begins to increase. There can be one guide or multiple guides who come to assist the student through a myriad of changes which will continue to happen throughout their life. As the word *guide* implies, they direct and clear the path traveled, not only for healing attributes, but for guidance on all aspects of life during an entire life span.

Most students find this attunement in Reiki reflects a far greater change than even the attunement within first degree. It often comes through re-evaluation of relationships with friends and associates, a better job and perhaps a new location to live. All of these changes are more in tune with the higher frequency of the body. When the apprentice changes, the world responds to the new, clearer vibration of the bodies: spiritual, mental, emotional and physical. It results in new perceptions created through the attunement.

The time following the attunement can bring on as many changes as the first attunement but, as the student begins to learn to easily adjust and flow with what life brings, the changes seem less intrusive. Peace is a part of Reiki and it allows one to transcend even the most difficult of issues with compassion and acceptance which make the change calmer. Clear awareness will allow gratitude to enter, as struggles become experiences which enrich life rather than stress it. Reiki practitioners can be noticed by others when they enter a room by the peaceful energy they radiate. They are found to be fully present with situations, empathetic, yet undisturbed, in their emotional fields.

The main differences of Reiki from other healing modalities are the intensity of the healing abilities and how it works on the students' personal growth. Individual advancement is stronger in Reiki than in other energy practices. Reiki opens a path which encourages the unleashing of the power within transcending what has been blocking personal growth in the past.

## The Etheric Bodies

Reiki is one of the easiest forms of healing around. In the course of asking for assistance, healing energy is granted. It is so simple and yet so profound. The energy flows through the practitioner and into the recipient through the clear intent to help. Without the knowledge of even the practitioner, the high healing vibration will enter the parts of the recipient's body where it is most needed. This includes all four bodies: the physical, mental, emotional and spiritual. Because Reiki works on all of these bodies, new perceptions as to why the recipient has an ailment are accessed.

Reiki and its symbols raise the vibration of all the bodies of the individual: physical, mental, emotional and spiritual. The physical body is the only one which is visible. The others are unseen, yet easily sensed. Prove it to yourself: notice how uncomfortable it feels when another person stands too close. This is because your personal space has been occupied without permission. This intruder has stepped into one of the three etheric bodies. There is no demarcation line to define this space, yet one is quite aware when another has crossed over this boundary. The invasion is within the spiritual, mental and emotional bodies. Reiki symbols increase the energy flow into these bodies by connecting to the universal energy which flows around the body thus increasing your awareness within these esoteric centers.

The **physical body** is where pain is recorded. This body is only a message center, directing one to the underlying reasons for distress originating in the subconscious. The **mental body** holds thoughts and if allowed to run unchecked, can cause physical disturbance. The **emotional body** is more covert. A great reference book to keep at hand is *Feelings Buried Alive Never Die* by Karol Truman. It is a start to understand what emotions lay dormant under a distressing physical problem. The **spiritual body**, though a connection to the higher aspect of the being, can still cause problems in the physical form. When the existence of this body is denied or ignored, this disconnect can manifest in emotional pain, which

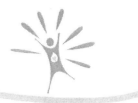

will eventually cause physical distress. This is not a religious awareness, rather it is a personal understanding of how gifts are given from the universe and how we return our gratitude for these accolades by using them or how we disregard them.

The heart center is very connected to the spiritual body. When this body is compromised the heart has difficulty receiving. Most of the dis-ease and pain in the energy fields of people or animals comes from a heart which is closed. The term
dis-ease is used to describe when the body is experiencing physical distress. The individual is not in the flow, thus uneasy with its current predicament, hence the term dis-ease.

Reiki is pure divine love and when administered without expectations the heart begins to understand it can open once again without feeling the pain of the past. Memories can arise but with a clearer perception than previously observed. There is no reason to fear these recollections, for the memory process is being guided by the divine self, through the transmission of Reiki.

It is in the blending and understanding of these four bodies that holistic health is achieved. Reiki brings in awareness and new observations to accomplish this goal.

To better understand dis-ease one must take time, become quiet and notice where the origin of the distressing sensation begins. The practice of meditation opens this pathway to understanding. The "Life Tools" listed in this book will assist the reader in accomplishing this goal.

"Life Tools" are guided imagery meditations which take the client deep into their subconscious mind where deep healing occurs. In hypnosis it is understood the subconscious mind rules the conscious mind. The conscious mind can analyze, command and direct, but it is the subconscious mind who is running the show. Tap into that part of the brain and the difference is apparent because the changes will then become permanent.

The act of giving Reiki takes the client deep into this part of the subconscious psyche. Notice how still your client becomes when you begin a treatment. This can also be observed during a self Reiki treatment.

**Example:** I notice when I access Reiki I feel like I am in an elevator going down but I am not moving, the down is coming into me. This "down sensation" is the Reiki. It immediately brings me into a place of stillness, my thoughts become silent and my body relaxed. I have a similar sense when I am hypnotized which tells me I am stepping into my subconscious mind with either process.

The practice of hypnosis, like Reiki, always leaves the client in charge. You are always in control, even if someone is guiding you and it is the same for Reiki. You make the decision to follow the guidance and you create and imagine the story which is revealed. With Reiki the energy enters the body and is guided to the appropriate place in the body by the guidance of the all knowing higher self. For *all* hypnosis is self-hypnosis and all healing is self healing.

The same is true when you are guiding your client with the guided imagery of a "Life Tool." The client takes control from the moment they enter the door. They share only the information they are ready to release at that time. This information gives permission to open doors to a clearer understanding through the process of Reiki. You become the guide and direct the client to places they have not looked before but they are the ones who see the imagery, intuit the information and create a new insight. This makes a much stronger bond to the truth, for they are not given new perceptions by the practitioner; they actually see and feel it for themselves.

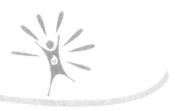

# Chapter 2

## Increasing the Power

As the practitioner channels Reiki energy regularly to themselves and others, their intuition will increase. This allows the practitioner to receive information about their client which is at first beyond the conscious awareness of either party. Not only does frequent use of Reiki increase inner knowing, it also can assist you as a therapist to connect to information from the higher self of their patron while treatments are being given. Often this information will not be gleaned until the time of the treatment but it can also come in earlier, sometimes as early as when the appointment is made.

The intuitive information received is not needed for Reiki to work, for Reiki is directed into the bodies of the receiver by the receiver's higher self. The knowledge and its use are given to the practitioner by the recipient's angels, guides or higher self, hence the simplicity of the work. Continued use of Reiki clears the channels to angels and guides of the recipient as well as the practitioner who is administering Reiki. This happens because the second degree Reiki attunement will square the healing energy acquired in the first degree attunement and vastly increase the intuition of the second degree Reiki practitioner.

Reiki is channeled from the universal life force energy that flows in and around the earth. It connects us to each other and to everything that is. The search for enlightenment and spiritual bliss often takes the seeker along many paths, but:

*~ What we seek is that which we are ~*

There is nothing outside of ourselves that cannot be found within the center of our being. In the search for our spiritual essence one might look for religions, practices, dogmas, gurus or masters. But the continued search for the thing that will make us perfect is futile, for what we seek is inherent and already attained, as it lies within our own hearts. Reiki opens the heart so that this knowledge can be found and most importantly, felt and shared. Once the student realizes this they can more easily allocate it to others. The increased power of Second Degree Reiki will augment this understanding.

## Symbols

Symbols have been used since the beginning of time to tell stories and to connect the physical to the divine. They are found throughout the world and can be seen in petroglyphs in Utah, hieroglyphs in Egypt and carvings on caves in Tibet, just to name a few. If you have ever stood by these writings you will attest to the feeling they emit. One can almost sense the spiritual nature of the artist. And yet the Reiki symbols have even more power than these geometric forms. This is because Reiki symbols radiate the light from the higher self, while other images receive their power from the conscious mind of those who have drawn them. It is still powerful but with a different focus.

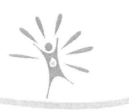

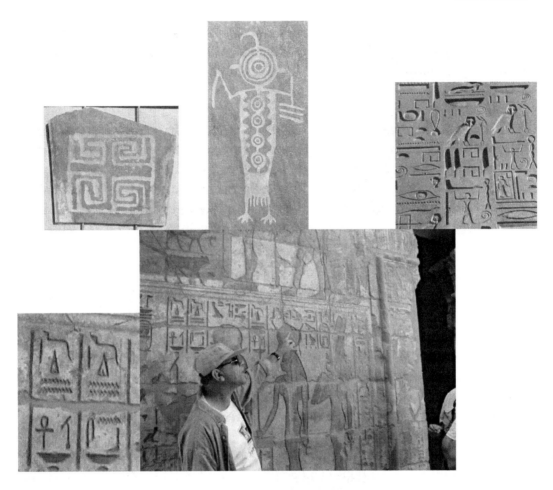

Petroglyphs and Hieroglyphs

Symbols are activated by vibrations, which can be through the sound of speaking the name of the symbol, through the act of drawing it or through simply holding the image in the mind. The movie *Contact* illustrates the concept of how sound, once put into the ethers, will never cease to exist. Jodie Foster plays a scientist who is fascinated with the exploration of contacting star systems as far away as humanly possible. After numerous attempts to receive a reply one signal is sent out and the response she receives is a 1940's newsreel broadcast. This is possible because radio and television frequencies are sound vibrations and once dispatched the vibrations of the sound will not stop; they continue into outer space for eternity.

Although *Contact* was a fictional story in the 1980's, there was an actual report of our astronauts receiving the transmission of an old radio broadcast when they were traveling out in space. Every verbal word has a vibration; once spoken, it continues to carry its intent forever. This is why avoiding detrimental words and speaking kindly is so important. Words carry their intention and amplify it whether they are negative or positive, so pay attention to your speech both audibly and the silent self talk within your mind.

## ~ *Words have power* ~

The vibrational energy of any image can be measured with a Radionics machine. This machine can broadcast frequencies to heal or to direct the wave lengths of an item into a location. It has been called "The Black Box" and it can access and adjust the subtle energy systems of people, animals, plants and objects. It has been set up to measure the vibration of lines or symbols on paper.

When the Reiki symbols were measured it was found that when they are drawn or spoken, their frequency and power are released. As with hands-on Reiki, the Reiki symbol itself emanates a very clear high frequency and when drawn, it combines with the energy of the practitioner and emits an even higher vibration. It then seeks out its counterpart in the universe, which intensifies its power once again. Once the symbol is drawn, it brings in the healing energy of anyone who has ever used that symbol, thus empowering healing through the symbol tremendously. This triple part sequence: the command of the practitioner, the influence of their higher self and support of anyone who has ever used these symbols, gives the symbol its overwhelming supremacy.

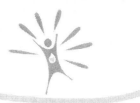

Reiki symbols do not work through the subconscious or physical mind, as do religious images. Reiki symbols connect to the mind of the higher self, thus moving beyond the limitations of the human mind and psyche. The symbol travels through space and time, much like prayer. Once activated with a stated intention it will no doubt manifest the appropriate result, because it is also amplified by the higher self of the recipient.

**Example:** After a period of practice, the symbols can be sent without drawing them by merely imagining them in your mind. When healing is sent the practitioner acts as a clear channel and the qualities of the symbols are then activated through their mind. The activity of drawing the symbol is a practice. Practice is defined as repeated performance or systematic exercise for the purpose of acquiring skill or proficiency. Once the student becomes accomplished in the drawing of the symbols, the skill is attained. The symbol is a tool. Once the energy of the form is embossed into the energy field of the practitioner through continued use, the drawing of the image becomes a preference rather than an absolute. This is how the healer steps into their power and away from the dogma of the symbol.

 **Remember:** Nothing is stronger than the divine gift of the individual healer: not the attunements, the symbols or the instruction.

All of these tools assist the seeker, but the power is already there, just dormant. The activity of drawing symbols and administering energy are merely a reminder of what lies within.

*~ Look within your heart for knowledge and power ~*

The attunement opens up the student to find and realize the gifts that have always been within. The purposes of the levels of Reiki are to allow this process to be gentle and new awareness to be observed. Some masters teach all levels of Reiki in one weekend, but this does not serve the student. When one rushes the process by experiencing all levels in only three days, much is lost. The student does not have time to integrate each level and become aware of how they effect their bodies: spiritual, mental and emotional. It is suggested that each level be separated by 21 days, this gives the student time to fully experience Reiki and how their bodies and chakras are being upgraded and cleansed. In this way a student can become a master in only three months; to some this may even appear to be the fast track. I honor my students' natural abilities to know when to proceed to the next level of Reiki. This allows them to choose how quickly they will progress in Reiki, for they are guided by their intuition and this knowing is one of the gifts of Reiki. My only request is that they give each level at least this 21 day integration period.

Step by step, with each degree of Reiki, the heart is opened and allowed to shine. This light within radiates out to others, showing the gifts they possess and their special healing attributes. Any dis-ease or pain is only the lack of love within and around the body. When you channel the love of Reiki any constructive desire becomes possible.

It is important to release any expectation of how the healing *should* occur. Too often one judges the results of their efforts by the effects obtained. Reiki works 100% of the time, even if no adjustments are apparent. Each physical and etheric body integrates the healing differently. The results may not always be sensed in the physical body. The mental, emotional and spiritual bodies are more personal in their content and the recipient may not share or even understand their observations pertaining to these changes.

The human form is a complex organism; therefore not all of the responses will be seen and understood immediately. Patience and trust, along with the ability to let go and move into the flow are paramount. An energy practitioner is not responsible for how the recipient receives and uses the force. We are free-will beings and that freedom must be given to all. Reiki will open the heart and bring

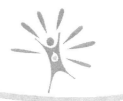

in new perspectives but the client gets to choose when to act on the information received. The changes may be sensed in the etheric bodies where the results are not visible to the physical or untrained eye. Be reassured that there are still changes happening. Trust the divine process of Reiki and do not judge the results or the lack thereof.

## Symbol Activation

Once the energy flow is commissioned, the connection is made and the energy transfer begins to channel from the higher self of the practitioner to the higher self of the receiver. The practitioner becomes a conduit of light and is blessed by the universal love which is streaming through. Translations have been made within the symbols for the learning styles of different societies. Consequently, the way the symbols are drawn is not critical. It is the desire to assist another which gives the symbols power, therefore your intent is most important. The guides understand the goal and follow the direction of the higher self of the recipient.

The attunement imprints the key of the symbol into the nervous system of the practitioner and activates the Reiki energy for the use of that symbol. The symbol does not have to be drawn perfectly to be recognized and activated by the spirit guides. Honor the symbol, draw it as accurately as possible, but do not become a perfectionist. Be clear in your mind as to what you want to accomplish and if it is of the highest good for the recipient, the request will be granted.

As the student advances, the symbols can be empowered simply with the conscious intent of its sender. The mind is a powerful instrument and, with practice, will activate the symbols without the tedious drawing of lines. This second degree healing develops the intuitive levels of the practitioner through practice. As the symbols are repeatedly drawn and memorized, the abilities of the initiate are increased on all levels in every facet of their life. Embrace the phrase "Practice makes perfect" for a time to honor the tradition of the symbol and then let go, allowing the natural tendencies of you, the practitioner to come through.

The divine is flowing in, so accept the energy of the symbols without question and notice how the symbol feels to you. Reiki is always about honoring the natural process which lies within each and every individual.

The instruction given in first degree Reiki revealed how the power symbol can be sent from the chakra in the palm of the hand or sent out the fire finger. The energy transferred from the palm can be wide and encompassing. When the fire

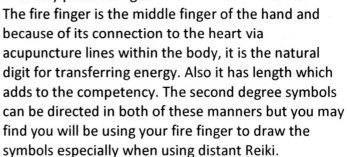

finger is used it becomes focused and intensely penetrating.

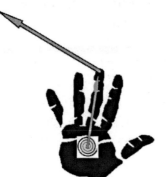

The fire finger is the middle finger of the hand and because of its connection to the heart via acupuncture lines within the body, it is the natural digit for transferring energy. Also it has length which adds to the competency. The second degree symbols can be directed in both of these manners but you may find you will be using your fire finger to draw the symbols especially when using distant Reiki.

## Cho-Ku-Rei

In most traditional Reiki teachings, Cho-Ku-Rei is a second degree symbol. Non-traditional Reiki teaches the power symbol in the initial class because it honors the advancement of humanity since the original teaching of Reiki in the early 1900's. The students during the current time period are ready for this energy of this symbol in their first class.

The Reiki power symbol is used to increase the energy in any given situation and also to seal a space in light and love. It has various uses and the sender has

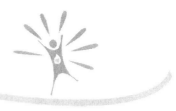

free will to add to this list and create their own. Try it out during your daily activities and keep track of the results. In this way, you will discover new possibilities, build your confidence in using symbol, as well as make your life flow with ease.

In the office, it can help to balance and harmonize meetings and discussions, and it can bring in new perceptions so the course of the entire day is harmonious. When problems arise Cho-Ku-Rei can calm irate customers, demanding bosses or difficult co-workers. Draw or imagine the form in a room, over the phone lines, on a desk or computer. Because Reiki channels a high frequency of energy, this symbol will bring in the power of love, which helps to harmonize any situation. It can even be used to direct clear perceptions into future meetings.

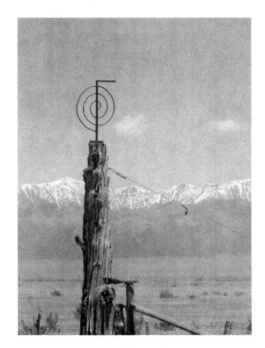 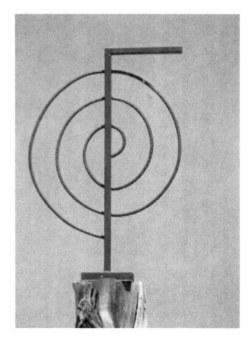

Cho-Ku-Rei over the
Colorado mountains

I found this Cho-Ku-Rei symbol on a ranch just outside of Crestone Colorado. Synchronicity was in play for I stopped to take the picture and at the same time the owner of the land drove up the county road. He was a delightful young man who traveled from Ohio with a friend to live their dream. This is a sustainable ranch which houses sheep, yaks, chickens, horses, organic crops and is supported by solar energy. Not surprisingly, these two young men were Reiki masters.

In the healing arena, Cho-Ku-Rei will direct more energy into a specific part of the body or bodies. When you start your Reiki treatments with Cho-Ku-Rei, the entire room will be sealed in light as well as the client and you as the practitioner. When used at the end of a treatment, it will ground the healing to the earth and allow the treatment to continue for days afterwards.

When traveling by air, turbulence can be avoided by imagining the symbol on the wings of the plane. The straight lines are drawn on the wings and the spiral appears to drop down a good distance, this will give the plane more mass, thus a larger, steadier form to fly through the rough weather. I find it rarely to fail.

Drawing Cho-Ku-Rei, the Power Symbol

Pronunciation:   (Cho koo ray)

Japanese translation

    Cho:   distance or length

    Ku:   able to remove suffering

    Rei:   steps toward inner peace

Begin drawing the symbol by starting at the right moving to the left, go straight down and make three clockwise circles, allowing each circle to encompass the previous while becoming smaller.

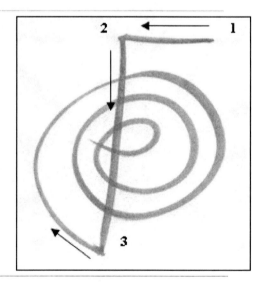

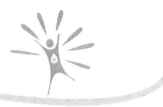

## Sacred Geometry with Cho-Ku-Rei

- The top line is drawn from right to left, representing the flow of male energy.
- The vertical line is drawn from top to bottom and is a reflection of energy extending from the cosmos to the earth and down the spinal column.
- The circle honors the female essence, the galaxy and the vital life force held in the spiral.
- All of the lines come together to form a balanced whole.
- Notice how the energetic flow of the spiral crosses the representation of the spinal column seven times, flowing through each of the seven chakras to open and balance them.

## How to use the Power Symbol

1. Cho-Ku-Rei is used to direct the energy of Reiki to a specific place.

2. Cho-Ku-Rei *turns on* the healing energy.

3. Cho-Ku-Rei opens the access channel to the love which surrounds all life, and activates a flow of cosmic light.

4. Cho-Ku-Rei is used before starting a treatment to seal the space in sacred luminescence.

5. Cho-Ku-Rei enfolds a room and enlightens the people involved, allowing for new perceptions in old situations.

6. Cho-Ku-Rei brings in a wall of protection between the recipient and the practitioner.

a. During the treatment, neither the client nor the practitioner absorbs the negativity or imbalances of the other.

b. When used at the end of a treatment, it grounds and completes the process.

c. When drawn over the solar plexus a ring of light is created around the recipient, locking the healing in for at least three days.

d. Healing energy is contained and absorbed by the recipient.

7. The benefits will be felt for three days after the treatment.

a. The energy felt on the day of treatment is primarily in the physical body.

b. The three succeeding days it will be noticed in the mental, spiritual and emotional bodies.

c. Inform the client of this extended process so they may receive the full benefit of their treatment.

8. Cho-Ku-Rei can be drawn at a doorway so whoever passes through will be blessed. Use in classrooms, office meetings, airplanes, hospital rooms, etc.

9. Imagine the symbol on the wings of an airplane to stop turbulence. The straight lines are over the wings and the spiral extends down to give the plane mass.

10. Use on airplanes at the entrance door, cockpit, galley, over engines at the wings and for anyone who is observed being upset in the plane.

11. Use in classrooms to hold the attention of young students or to aid an instructor so they will present information in a clear concise manner.

12. Use at office meetings for focus, understanding, power in their prescribed field and cooperation.

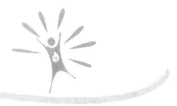

## Cho-Ku-Ret

Pronunciation:  (Cho Koo Ret)
Non-traditional Symbol   (used to empower inanimate objects)

Cho-Ku-Ret has no power on its own, therefore sandwich it between the power of two Cho-Ku-Rei's. Use it only on objects, as this is where it holds its power.     Cho-Ku-Rei brings power into living things as Cho-Ku-Ret is for non-life forms. First draw a Cho-Ku-Rei then Cho-Ku-Ret and finish with another Cho-Ku-Rei. This symbol has a lovely flow to it. Those of you who loved the old TV sitcoms of the 70's may recall how to draw this symbol by remembering the "L" worn by Laverne in "Laverne and Shirley." Imbedded in the symbol you will see Laverne's "L" or imagine a scripted "L."

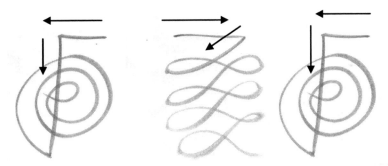

Cho Ku Ret:
1. May be used on candles to emphasize the light they are bringing into a situation or room.
2. Use to enhance efficiency of computers.
3. Aids in the mechanical running of a car or other machinery.
4. It will augment the performance of musical instruments.

5. Use on golf clubs, golf balls, roller blades, bicycles, skis and other sports equipment to balance and align the object to the body.

## Cho-Ku-Ret   Alternate Variation

An alternative symbol has been created which is simple and faster to draw yet still embraces the same energies of the original image. This symbol does not need Cho-Ku-Rei on either side, as Cho-Ku-Rei is already incorporated into it. Either variation of the symbol will bring the same result.

Begin by drawing part of Cho-Ku-Rei and, as you start the second circle, make an infinity symbol in the center.

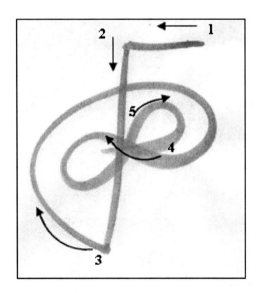

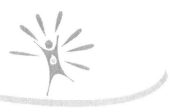

# Chapter 3

## The Mental and Emotional Symbol

The mental and emotional symbol will gently bring to the surface the buried issues which need to be addressed and cleared. Because this is a Reiki symbol, it holds the intelligence of the higher self and will not bring up more than the client can handle at the time. If an old memory has been stimulated, the client is ready to address it and is supported by his/her guides in facing it. The awareness of the old issue will come in with an entirely new perspective than has been seen in the past, and of course, embraced with love.

This symbol has a myriad of uses which will help with relationships of all kinds: personal, business, family and romantic. Energy cords can be released and neutral spaces can be created for conversation and confrontations. Spirits can be released to move on to the light. The processes will be supported by the "Life Tools" found in the following chapter.

## Sei-He-Ki , The Mental and Emotional Symbol

Pronunciation: (Say Hay Key)

Translation:
   Bringing in new perceptions through the process of thought and a new awareness in the feelings.

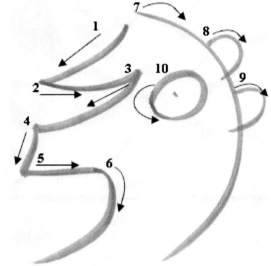

   Sei:
      A state, like a growing stage of being
      Things hidden inside
      The origin of external form
   He Ki:
      Japanese word for "root chakra"
      Off balance
      A strange partiality
      Balance the things hidden off-balance inside
      Resonates to potential harmony

If you can imagine a familiar picture within the symbol it will make drawing the symbols much easier and aid in remembering the image. In Sei-He-Ki one might see a dragon, pig or the number five. Allow your imagination to direct you to a recognizable form to help you recall this symbol. The numbering system of the symbols also aids in its memorization.

The symbol may be drawn with your hand in the air in front of your body, over the body of the recipient, or written on paper to enhance healing and affirmations. The intent of its use is more important than how precisely it is drawn, but be as exact as you can to honor the symbol. Most of all, have a clear heart and the intent to help another out of emotional or mental distress. This will strengthen the power coming from the symbol.

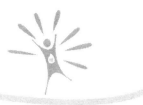

 **Remember:** This is a tool; *you* are the channel of the love it emits.

## How to use the Mental and Emotional Symbol

Sei-He-Ki will locate the core issue attached to emotional distress that is affecting the physical body and heal that aspect of one's life. Sometimes a new perspective will be obtained when thinking about a distressing event from the past. If it is not fully integrated, it will resurface in a different way until the full knowledge is acquired. Therefore ask for the core incident to surface. When a situation is seen through the eyes of love and not fear or judgment, it is seen in an entirely new light. Once the original incident is cleared through the activation of love, the subsequent incidents will drop like dominos. Sei-He-Ki will make this process less painful than conventional methods because Reiki is pure divine love and the issue does not need to be readdressed.

Not only can Sei-He-Ki be used for emotional well being, but it can be used for mental enhancement as well. It can help improve memory, locate lost objects, assist in learning new concepts and balance the left and right hemispheres of the brain for whole brain cognition.

Lost items can be found in two ways. The first way is to become still and draw Sei-He-Ki while waiting for intuitive direction to surface. The energy of Reiki, brought in through the activation of this symbol, will relax the mind, allowing memories to surface.

The other is to call upon a divine being that is proficient in the process of locating lost articles. His name is Cyclopea, considered to be "the all seeing eye of God." His image is found within the pyramid on the back of the United States dollar bill. His retreat on earth is in the Teton Mountains in Wyoming. Ask for His assistance and your misplaced piece will magically appear.

Have you ever questioned why there is a pyramid with Cyclopea's eye on the back of a dollar bill? The answer could lie within the history of our nation's founding fathers. Many of them were known to be members of the secret order of the Masonic Lodge. This was an esoteric group who believed in the powers of the optimistic thought, ascended masters, like Cyclopea, and our ability to manifest positive situations and actions with the aforementioned. The pyramid and the eye of Cyclopea reflect this possible connection.

Because Sei-He-Ki is a mental symbol as well as an emotional one, it can be a treasure when new concepts are being presented. It will bring clarity of thought along with clear understanding and an intuitive sense on how to best apply the new found information. Often when new ideas arise, there is some hesitation before proceeding to the next step. One might not trust the process or expect it to work for them. The use of Reiki opens doorways and illumines the path so the new idea can come to fruition.

When using the symbols, the mental process will also be enhanced when both hemispheres of the brain are activated and balanced. Place your hands on either side of your head or the client and imagine Sei-He-Ki. Through the healing process the brain will begin to integrate.

Develop a sense of non-attachment to the results of the energy treatment. What appears to have no effect could be working in ways not yet discovered. In the event of an abusive relationship, when the symbol Sei He Kei is used and the unhealthy relationship still continues, know that light is filling the spiritual, emotional and mental bodies of the parties involved. It may take time for the results to become apparent, as the physical body integrates the process and acts on it.

Reiki works 100% of the time. Know that if a person continues to stay in the same abusive relationship, it is probably the safest place for them to be at that time. If they have not yet been empowered to understand why they chose this experience in life, they might find yet another abusive partner and the next one

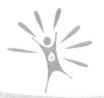

may inflict more abuse than they or their family members can handle. Know that Reiki always works for the highest and best good for the parties involved. Be unattached to the results and trust that the divine knowledge of Reiki is in charge, assisted by love.

Apply the model given and see which works best for you. Nothing is written in stone, there is not just one way to accomplish any feat. Our personal energies vary and resonate differently. Honor your individuality, play with the symbols and concepts presented and then make your own decision as to the best way to proceed with the symbols in a treatment.

When to Use Sei-He-Ki:

1. Use to address and bring to the surface the core issues and original cause of any given disturbance, physical, mental or emotional.
2. Use as a spiral of protection around the body.
   a. See the mental and emotional symbol as a circular form encompassing the body. Draw it in front of you as large as your body and step into it.
   b. This will harmonize the feelings and protect one from outside influences.
3. Use to improve memory. Visualize Sei-He-Ki, relax and thoughts will float to the surface of the mind.
4. Use to find lost objects. Use Sei-He-Ki or Cyclopea to instill an answer.
   a. Imagine Sei-He-Ki while commanding the illusive item to reappear.
   b. Call to the ascended master Cyclopea, the all seeing eye of God and ask for His assistance in locating the article.
   c. Use a pendulum along with the symbol to track and find the piece. Pendulum instruction is found in Chapter six.
5. Use to aid in understanding literature or taking tests.

a. Draw the mental and emotional symbol on the book or test.

b. Hold the papers between your hands.

c. Send Reiki into the document; take a few deep breaths and your mind will clearly receive the information being presented.

6. If you are confused at a lecture or class, use these techniques:

a. Place your hands on your legs; send the symbol to yourself and to the facilitator.

b. If you do not understand the information, it could be the instructor's inability to disseminate information; often you are not at fault. Send Reiki to the presenter to assist them organizing their thoughts and getting back on track.

7. Apply Sei-He-Ki while studying, to integrate the right and left hemispheres of the brain for integrated learning, increased comprehension and whole brain activation.

a. Left side of brain is the thinking, linear, analytical part of the mind.

b. Right side of brain is where our creative and imaginative mind processes lie.

c. Very helpful to balance the confusion of dyslexia.

8. Use in relationships, whether business, family or intimate partners

a. The relationship holds its own form, similar to a third person or another entity.

b. Send Sei-He-Ki to that entity.

c. You cannot control people with this symbol.

d. It works only for the highest good for all concerned.

e. Relationships may need to transform and break up for growth.

f. Reiki will assist in a harmonious and healthy release.

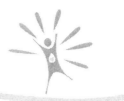

## Balancing the Right and Left Brain

There are time when the information received is not adequate to make a clear decision. One must then use deductive reasoning along with intuition in order to choose the appropriate action. Thinking in this way uses the rational left brain and the instinct of the right brain simultaneously. Many people use only one side of their brain at a time which will not allow clear information to be processed. By drawing Sei-He-Ki, one will pull information from both sides of the brain in a balanced manner. The results can be astounding. You may try this visual exercise to experience the sensation of working with whole brain thinking for yourself.

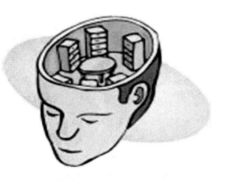

The Left Brain
- Logical
- Sequential
- Rational
- Analytical
- Objective
- Look at parts

To access the knowledge in the left brain imagine becoming so small that you can picture yourself sitting inside the frontal lobes of your brain. This is all done with visual imaging. Start by moving to the left side of your head and imagine a room. Place in this space what sustains the thoughts which run in your mind. There could be books, manuals, computers, televisions and/or newspapers. Thoughts dominate your thinking in this part of your head and everything here needs to be analyzed completely. Keep this process going until you really get a sense of this type of deductive reasoning, then notice how it makes you feel. Are you apprehensive, nervous or comfortable? Just pay attention and observe your reactions.

The Right Brain
- Random
- Intuitive
- Holistic
- Creative
- Subjective
- Looks at whole rather than parts

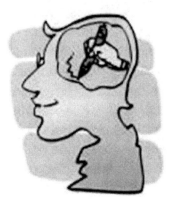

Imagine standing up and walking from the left side of your brain over to the right side and create what that might look like. This is the sensory part of your thinking. To get in touch with this section of your thinking process, you will need to imagine you are tangibly becoming aware of your feelings. You will be activating this section of the brain by awakening all five senses: sight, touch, hearing, smell and taste.

Visualize a soft red velvet chair and sit on it; feel its texture as you run your hand along the cloth. It is soft when you move your hand in one direction and resistant and rough when your hand slides in the opposite way. There is a window to your right. Sense the warmth of the sunlight streaming in, feel the coolness of the breeze on a summer day, smell the sweet scent of flowers wafting through the window. The flower smells so sweet you can almost taste it. You are now in contact with your five senses. This will begin to open your intuition as you allow your mind to wander and pick up new thoughts.

While in the right side of the brain become aware of how you feel emotionally, physically and mentally. Compare it to how you felt in the left side of your brain. Which side is more comfortable or familiar? From the sensations perceived, can you tell where you spend most of your time in your thought process, knowing there is no correct place to be?

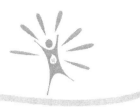

In this calm state of new awareness, in the intuitive part of your mind, after accessing all the knowledge you have gleaned from the left side of your brain, guidance will open and answers will appear. Notice the way you perceive the information; it may be a picture, a sense or just an inner knowledge you were not aware of previously. The information may not come to mind until later that day, when you least expect it. It could be when you are doing mindless work: walking, showering, listening to music, just as you are falling asleep or as you are waking up in the morning. These are calm states when perceptions can float up into consciousness. Be open, relaxed and trust that the information will come to you.

**Example:** There are occasions when direction comes through while I am in the shower, while other times my problem solving will come to me in the middle of the night. I awake long enough to receive the answer to my question and then I fall back to sleep. In years past, I was afraid I would forget my inspiration so I would write down the incoming response before I fell back asleep. I have now learned the information once grasped is mine to keep and it is always there in my consciousness when I awake in the morning. Just begin to pay attention to your thoughts, write them down, and with this practice, more will arise.

You have learned how to perceive whether you are working from the right or left brain but the ultimate process is to integrate and use both sides of the brain simultaneously. Try this exercise to move into whole-brain thinking: after contacting the right and left brain in the previous exercise, create a picture of sitting in the dividing hemisphere of your brain. Notice if there is a barrier in this space. What keeps you from easily traversing from your analytical mind to your creative thoughts? Is it a brick wall which needs to be demolished, a curtain which requires opening, or a window that could be cleaned to reveal information? This is your imagery. If you see nothing, make up a story, create a picture and then remove it.

**Remember:** It is a scientific fact that the mind does not know the difference between imagination and reality. The brain waves are the same whether you envision a situation or if it is actually happening.

So don't think pretending is a childish practice and nothing can come of it. You are entraining your brain to recall intuitive imagery and it will respond. If you pretend there is no separation between the right and left hemispheres of your brain, your consciousness will then become one integral part. From this state you can easily access the deepest part of your creativity while staying connected to the analytical intelligence which you have fostered during this lifetime. The following "Life Tool" may be administered in a self treatment or for a client.

 Life Tool: Whole Brain Integration

| | |
|---|---|
| 1. | Sit comfortably in a quiet place. Take three deep, slow cleansing breaths. |
| 2. | Allow tension to release from your body with each exhalation. |
| 3. | Imagine yourself becoming so small you could walk into your brain. |
| 4. | Direct your attention to the left side of your brain. |
| 5. | Design a room for your thinking mind; include: |
| | a. Books, papers, pencils and former experiences. |
| | b. Computers and research materials. |
| 6. | Get a sense of the analytical process of the mind. |
| | a. How does it feel when you are in this mode? |
| | b. Are you anxious, apprehensive, stressed or comfortable? |
| | c. Remain here until you are fully aware of the sensations created when working from the left brain. |
| 7. | After this realization, pretend to move over to the right side of your |

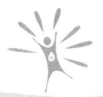

| | brain. This is a place where you will awaken all five of your senses. |
|---|---|
| 8. | Imagine a large red velvet chair and sit in it. |
| | a. Feel the tactile sensation of soft velvet. |
| | b. Allow your body to sink into the comfortable cushion as it envelops your body. |
| 9. | There is an open window to your right. Feel the warmth of the sunlight on your body, a breeze wafting over your skin. |
| 10. | Allow a gentle breeze to blow your hair across your face as you notice the scent of flowers so sweet you can almost taste them. |
| 11. | Contact the feeling of being in the right brain and notice if this is a comfortable place to reside. |
| 12. | Move to the center hemisphere of your brain. Remove any imaginary barriers between the right and left brain so you may access whole brain thinking. |
| 13. | Let your mind wander and be open to receiving new ideas emitted in the breeze from mother earth. |
| 14. | Notice how your mind receives thoughts. |
| | a. Watch to see if they come in pictures, sensations or feelings. |
| | b. An inner knowledge is being awakened. |
| | c. The brain is now balanced and new ideas will be floating to the surface. |
| 15. | Imagine how you will place your ideas into action from this newly created space. Relax and know you are now in the flow. |
| 16. | When you feel complete, take a deep breath and open your eyes. |
| 17. | More information will be available to you during the next three days, so expect it. |

## Healing Relationships

Relationships can be defined within the parameters of personal, business and family. The most important is the connection to self, for if this is out of sync, no matter how hard you try, you will not be able to create a balance with anyone else. This is why self Reiki treatments are so vital to a fulfilled life. There can be times when we interact with others and become triggered, which stimulate old issues within the physical, mental and emotional bodies. When any of these bodies become over-charged and unbalanced there can be trouble communicating.

Reiki continually pours love into all four bodies thus stabilizing them. This keeps the attention away from blaming others for our struggles and focusing on any of their negative attributes. Because Reiki is pure divine love, with the use of Sei-He-Ki, most turmoil within the personal framework of relationships can be understood, blessed and appeased in a gentle and compassionate manner. Sei-He-Ki will enlighten the user to new perceptions and release any judgments out of the energy fields.

One way to better understand a situation and let go of stressful confrontations and memories is by giving the mind a tangible image to focus upon. A relationship space in the form of a sphere will become that figure. This bubble will hold opinions and ideas of others so you will not harbor them in your bodies.

Create a 12 inch bubble out in front of you. This we will call the relationship space. Extend a tube from your heart into this sphere and fill it with love. The bubble should be outside of your aura, which would be about 18 inches from your body.

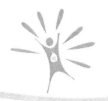

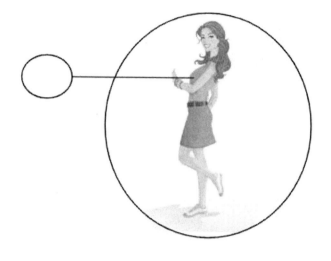

Creating the
relationship space

Place others' ideas into this space so they may be observed without feeling a need to quickly make a decision. This can be done for individuals as well as groups. Here the concepts can be analyzed without emotion and one can come to better conclusions.

When one feels drained or agitated after a discussion, it is because the words expressed were not allowed to stay in the relationship space. It was taken in personally and allowed to fester within the aura, usually in the mental and emotional bodies. This clouds the perception and one might make a decision which is not in their best interest. Once the ideas of others have been removed from the body and aura and placed in the relationship bubble, notice how it feels. There should be a sense of relaxation.

To clear any disturbances out of your body and energy fields, think of the words which were expressed during a conversation along with any emotions. Give them a color and texture to make the memory solid in the mind. Next, track where these issues are residing. Are they in the aura (mental turmoil and emotions) or physical body (pain or discomfort)? Imagine them moving out of the body, through the aura and into the relationship space. Do the same for the other party by removing the imposed thoughts and feelings you directed into them. From this vantage point, the annoyance may be observed without personal feelings becoming charged.

If these images are negative and not necessary for the harmonious completion of the given situation, allow them to drain down into the earth. From the center of the relationship bubble extend a cord down into the earth and let the contrary feelings be released. Mother Earth will not hold onto the negativity. She will actually neutralize it with love.

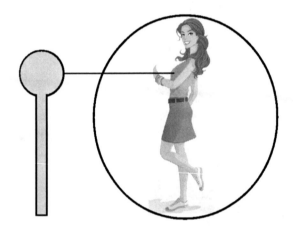

Grounding negative emotions and conversations to the earth

To expedite the process of grounding out negativity, imagine divine light flowing into the top of the relationship space while the negativity is releasing out of the bottom. The process will then move faster. This is called an "energy transfer." To stimulate the senses assign different colors to what is being released and what is brought in. The more the senses are activated the greater will be your success. Do not blindly believe what I tell you; notice what you experience by using the following "Life Tool."

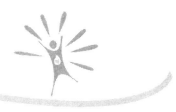

 Life Tool:  Clearing Space with an Energy Transfer

| |
|---|
| 1. Recall a situation when you felt pushed to make a quick decision or agitated by the words, actions or opinions of another person or group of people. |
| 2. In your mind's eye, create a 12-inch bubble, 18-inches out in front of your body. |
| 3.  Within your aura or body are the words, feelings and opinions of another person. Give these thoughts a color and texture. |
| 4. Push the energy and ideas of the other party out of your aura and into the relationship bubble. |
| 5. Do the same for the other party by removing the imposed thoughts and feelings you directed into them. |
| 6. This will give you the opportunity to observe their concepts from a neutral space, unencumbered by their personal agenda. |
| 7. Notice if you feel different about their ideas when these concepts reside in this neutral space rather than in your body. |
| 8. If any concepts are negative, release them from the bottom of the bubble. |
| 9. Place a grounding cord in the center of the relationship space and create a path for adversity to drain out. |
| 10. Give the energy a color and allow any opposing thoughts to move into the earth to be neutralized by the loving light of mother earth. |
| 11. Simultaneously, imagine divine light entering the top of the relationship space as it pushes out any negativity. |
| 12. This energy transfer will expedite the cleansing process, leaving the relationship space a clear loving place with space for new more harmonious concepts to be perceived. |

Sacred geometry is the study of patterns which have been found throughout the world, dating far back in time, probably as long as humans have inhabited the earth. In sacred geometry, correlations are made between what seem to be average images in our lives and then are perceived as divine interactions because they transform energies around us. They are considered sanctified because their forms continue to be repeated in nature from the numeric patterns of flower petals to the specific ratio of the spirals found in a ram's horns and seashells. You can even see references to these sacred geometric forms in the movie *The Da Vinci Codes*. Although the story is fictitious, it refers to the Catholic Church and ancient understandings of how such forms have been adapted.

Since the beginning of time, symbols have been used to represent the spiritual understandings and stories of societies. They are still prevalent today, etched on stone walls, found in books and represented in art. Even though they have aged, the energy from these images can still be sensed, for they were hallowed forms drawn to reflect the sacredness that lies within the human spirit.

The relationship space can also be compared to one of these ancient geometric symbols, the Vesica Pisces. This is a form which was long ago adopted by religions and referred to as the bladder of the fish. Its origins started long before the concept of Christianity and was used by many primitive tribes and medieval artists throughout the world. The Vesica Pisces can be imagined as another place which can be a safe haven for relationships.

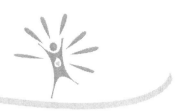

## Vesica Pisces

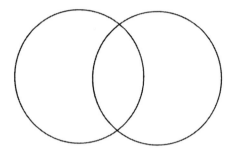

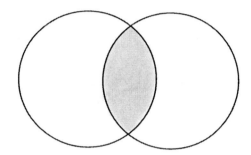

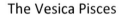

The Vesica Pisces                    The center holds
mysterious powers

The Vesica Pisces is comprised of two overlapping spheres which then create a center with mysterious powers. This intersection has had numerous interpretations by various cultures and religions. It is no wonder its form has been seen over the years in medieval churches throughout Europe. In the Middle Ages its real meaning was kept secret because it reflected a source of immense power and energy. The powers to be at that time did not feel the people could handle such a force. Perhaps Renaissance artists hid this form in their art and architecture to secretly empower the people.

Christians call the center area, the bladder of the fish partly because one can envision a fish in the center, as is shown in the following image. This correlates to Christianity because Jesus was known as a fisherman of souls. To help the native people accept the new religious dogma, images were used which were familiar to them thus making Christianity appear to not be as foreign to their spiritual makeup.

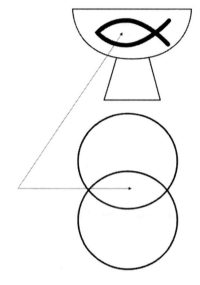

From the Vesica Pisces
emerges the Christian Icon
the bladder of the fish

Vision comes not only from our physical eyes, but also from the third eye in the forehead called our inner sight which we use while meditating. Using the power of the center of the Vesica Pisces while meditating can increase intuitive powers and the intent of the meditation. Focusing on this image while talking with another person will activate loving energy, increasing the harmonious intent of the conversation. When concepts are placed into this form and allowed time to process, new ideas will immerge.

Mutual Understanding Space

Another way to look at the relationship space is by using the center of the Vesica Pisces to house the relationship energies. Imagine two overlapping circles encompassing each individual. The center will be the mutual understanding space. In order to stabilize a relationship only one partner needs to be consciously aware of this form and have a clear intent for harmony and balance. In this field, truth can be spoken void of fear, because both individuals will feel the love this space holds. Thoughts are often more clearly understood when there is no personal

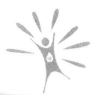

energy clouding the words, by placing the dialogue in the center space, this clarity will be accomplished.

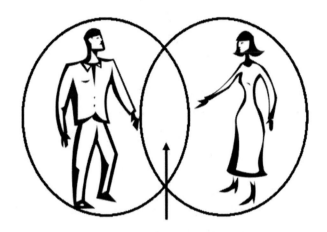

Neutral energy is held in the mutual understanding space

To ease stress after conflicting conversations with family members, friends, or business associates, imagine a sphere of energy around the parties involved, enveloping each person and their ideas. The center is an energized, holy place where the heart easily resides. With the intent to make this a location for the peace in the heart, so it becomes. This works for groups as well as individuals. The Vesica Pisces can help in business meetings by placing an individual in one circle and the group in the other. When you do this days before the rendezvous you will see how much better ideas will flow.

This is similar to the energy created with the energy bubble used previously in healing relationships. The bubble is good to use in the moment during or after a conversation. This keeps the influence of another from clouding your true desires. The process using the Vesica PIsces can be used when you need an idea to "cook", which allows the flavors of the input of others to blend and enhance the entire concept.

An individual can become attached to their own ideas and suggestions thus clouding their perception of other ideas during business or personal matters. The attachment to the outcome can create a sense of control, thus making friends or colleagues resistant to even hearing another's idea. In the center of the Vesica Pisces, suggestions are laid upon a clear ground that is free of conditions. It is a concept offered for consideration with no desire to control the outcome. When a concept is presented from a personal space rather than a mutual understanding space, there could be old patterns attached to how it is perceived. When an idea is presented in the mutual understanding space, there is less chance of being misunderstood.

In this area, it is easy to be impartial to another's opinion without taking the information presented personally. Because this is a space of heart, it holds the ability for you to express truth while the corresponding person is not feeling that your ideas are being pushed upon them. Any judgments or emotions stay in the center and are not absorbed into either personal sphere. Because of this, one can be compassionate without being drained of energy. Each individual will feel heard and acknowledged because of the empathy held within this form.

Patterns of communication with family members are established early in our youth. These blueprints can be difficult and uncomfortable to break if not approached with care. Working from the heart is the key. As you make changes in how you are reacting to others, family members may become upset. They expect you to play the role created within the old family patterns and when you don't, it can create a riff. This can be unfamiliar territory for not only you, but for them as well.

Our greatest fear is the fear of the unknown and others' negative reactions come from this fear as well. As one becomes assured and empowered in their new image, they will find that their family and partners will adjust to their way of being and become more harmonious. Be patient as you wait for this to happen and as you hold your own.

There is a kindness which radiates from the mutual understanding space and that is why intimate partners will relax when this space is formed during conversations even though they might be unaware you have created it.

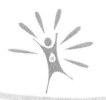

Remember in confrontations, it is your reaction to another that creates the resistance. As you release the attachment to the outcome, the charge is then neutralized. You may do this by placing thoughts and ideas into the mutual understanding space to defuse the energy, allowing new co-creative ideas to emerge.

> **Example:** The childhood game tug of war, aptly illustrates the power of letting go. In the game, each team holds a rope and tries to pull the other team over a line. If one side would drop the rope the resistance would be released and the other team would drop to the ground. The same holds true in resistant conversations, if there is no resistance the issue would be dropped.

When presenting an idea, place it in the center of the Vesica Pisces so others will not feel controlled by your suggestion and they can draw their own conclusions without your influence. Conversing in this space will be advantageous, as it alleviates the charge when another has trouble understanding the concepts presented or appears to invalidate your ideas. This space allows one to feel more aligned after an intense discussion.

When conflicts arise, the first response is often to send Reiki to the individual who appears to be creating the disturbance. This process can hold judgment toward the actions of the other.

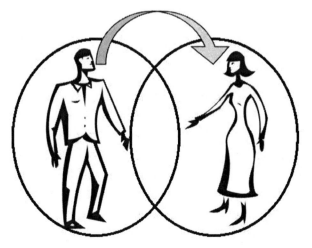

Directing Reiki to
another person

When Reiki is sent into the mutual understanding space, new perceptions are activated while deeper healings are occurring. Reiki is energy which will be felt on many and often subtle levels. When Reiki is sent into a common space of love, it becomes fertile ground where new concepts can germinate and grow, bringing new observations for all involved.

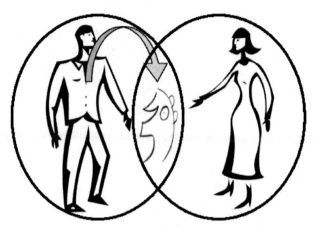

Directing Reiki into the mutual understanding space

When no conclusion can be reached in a business meeting or personal conversation, suggest the situation be set aside until a future time. In the mean time place the information presented by all parties in the space of the Vesica Pisces. It then resides in a nurturing space and has the opportunity to blend with the ideas of each person involved. When looking into the form the proposals combine and may appear to take on a color or picture as they are released into the center space. This now holds the possibility for new thoughts to be obtained by all the individuals involved.

With everyone's ideas in the imaginary of the Vesica Pisces, have the intention that these thoughts are becoming building blocks for new concepts. Plan a time to revisit the information, perhaps in a few days, and you just may be surprised at the results. Over a period of time, new models will arise from the combined energy of all involved. Any one individual on their own would not have found these ideas, but when the enigma is allowed time to process in this space of divine love, new plans appear. This is the beauty of using this process; it is simple.

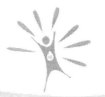

Nothing needs to be done, other than placing the exchange in this sacred space and giving it time to intertwine with the thoughts of another. Love will do the rest.

**Example:** In one of my classes there was a married couple who took second and third degree Reiki together. Upon the start of the third degree class the husband shared that he had used Sei-He-Ki in the mutual understanding space as instructed in the second degree class. He came to the conclusion that the marriage was no longer serving either one of them. When I asked his wife how she felt about his decision, she was not in agreement. I continued to question her about how she saw the marriage as I sent Reiki love to her through my eyes.

During a mini counseling session she expressed that over the 15 years of their marriage she had not found time to pursue her love of art and also missed living by the ocean. In only an hour she could see how their marriage was not serving either one of them and this break up was mutually beneficial. Once she let go of how things "should" be she became comfortable with the idea of how leaving each other would create a new, more balanced life apart.

Reiki did not split up their marriage; Reiki opened them to realize how their lives could be fuller and more loving if they were apart. Reiki always works 100% of the time but it might not be in the way we first perceive in our minds.

*~ It is in letting go of expectations that we become free ~*

In this exercise the Vesica Pisces will be seen as a common ground, a shared vision and a place of mutual understanding. The power held in this area is pure love. When focusing on this area a person will be able to hold to their individual ideas while safely speaking their truth. Others involved will relax, sensing there is a safe space which has been created to converse where they too may express their ideas honestly without fear of judgment. This happens because the form holds compassion, respect and truth through love.

Life Tool: Mutual Understanding Space

The process of using the mutual understanding space can involve two parties or groups of people. The two circles of the Vesica Pisces will encompass the opposing parties and at their intersection will be the power of the Vesica Pisces, the area of understanding and love.

| | |
|---|---|
| 1. | Develop a sphere around your body in your mind's eye. |
| 2. | Imagine an equal sphere around the body of the person or group you are conversing with. |
| 3. | Allow the spheres to overlap and create a Vesica Pisces. |
| 4. | Place the ideas expressed in the area in the center of the form. |
| 5. | This holds the heart energy where there is no judgment of any of the concepts presented. |
| 6. | When presenting your ideas, place them in the center of the Vesica Pisces so others will not feel controlled by your presentation. |
| 7. | As the conversation proceeds, let their reply stay in the center space; do not let their words and emotions enter into your personal sphere. |
| 8. | From the area of your personal sphere, you may integrate and process their concepts without being influenced by their opinions. |
| 9. | All parties involved will feel heard and validated in this space. |
| 10. | When conclusions cannot be made during conversations, allow all ideas to stay within the center space and meld for a time. |
| 11. | Revisit the discussion in a few days. |
| | a. The center is fertile ground. |
| | b. Ideas will converge and grow. |
| | c. New concepts will be created and will be a combination of each person's ideas. |
| 12. | New ideas will have formed over time and can be accessed by both |

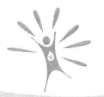

| parties. |
|---|
| 13. This will make a balanced, co-creative relationship. |

## Using Affirmations

Affirmations are one way to empower your desires and become more self-sufficient. But how do statements alone improve your life? Can these changes be made by sheer will alone? No. Sheer will comes from the conscious mind, as do many affirmations. It is only when we enter the subconscious mind that we make a lasting change. Use Sei-He-Ki and ask for access into the subconscious mind as you make your testimony. The power behind the words comes in the emotions which radiate from the heart. Reiki calms the bodies and through this will integrate the affirmation into the subconscious mind where permanent change occurs.

Positive statements can be anchored into the subconscious mind with guided imagery during deep meditation. Learning how to become deeply relaxed will assist in the positive effect of an affirmation. Reiki will aid in this process as Reiki activates the subconscious mind.

 **Remember:** Always use affirmative expressions.

Create your affirmations with positive language, for the universe will not respond to or recognize the negative form. If you say, "I will not eat chocolate," the universe will only hear, "I will eat chocolate." Not that this is a bad thing; it just may not be reflecting your first intention.

If you say, "I want more money" you will always "want" for money. Words have power, be cognizant of what you are expressing in the literal sense. When asking for money include all aspects of what money represents. Stay open to the different ways supply may show up in your life. If one only asks for currency, the other options may be lost. Finding someone who will trade for services is creating no need for money at all which is also a form of affluence. Trading time for money not only supplies but allows one to honor the attributes of another. And by knowing how to do Reiki you have a valuable gift to offer others.

When you require financial gain affirm, "I am grateful for my unlimited supply of every good thing." Unlimited supply opens your energy to receive in a myriad of ways not just monetarily. One can make more money just by finding reasonable prices on goods and services. Be open to receiving help from people you have yet to meet. A stranger could lay laurels at your feet, but if you only asked for money, you may need to work a long time to receive the same gift.

 **Remember:** Do not ask, affirm.

Now let's fine-tune the statement of asking. If you request to have something in your life, you are negating your power to manifest it. Make your request an affirmation of fact. Establish you already have what you are seeking, because you do. It is already in your energy field, all that is required is the acceptance of its presence in your physical arena.

 **Remember:** Give the affirmation as if it already happened.

Structure the statement of intent to reflect three time periods: the asking, the receiving and the gratitude. Even if you do not totally believe the statement you are making, still affirm its existence in your life. The best way to accomplish this is to be grateful for what you are asking for, even if you do not have it yet. As you move beyond the asking into receiving, the gratitude arises. Anchor your statement with a heartfelt emotion and your intention is on its way to fulfillment.

 **Remember:** Emotions have power.

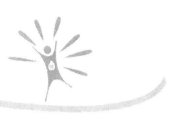

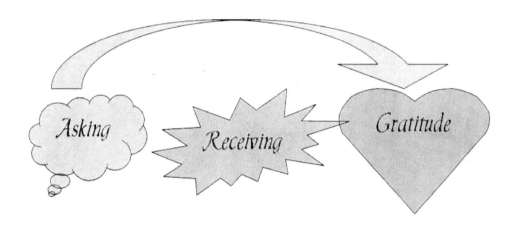

Save Steps – Move from asking directly to gratitude

Step into how it feels to have your desire in order to give it power. Emotions are what fuel your desire and they can have positive or negative energy. If you feel your desire is impossible to receive, it will be so. Once you empower your statement with a positive feeling it will increase the possibilities tenfold. When an affirmation is given, release it out into the Universe and accept its presence in your life. This allows you to receive all structures of wealth, even ones you could not imagine on your own.

Some find repeated affirmations work best to lock the desire into the sub-conscious mind. Another way to create the same effect is to make the statement once, with deep feeling, see it as a completed image and let go of it. Imagine your affirmation in a ball of energy, floating in the Universe. Rather than repeating the affirmation, merely check in on the request later to see how it is advancing. Look into the ball and see if anything has changed. It could be different in color and/or brightness, or its distance from you might have increased or decreased. Be assured your divine self is in charge making the appropriate adjustments.

Holding onto a declaration and saying it repeatedly can deny its manifestation. Sound is a living organism, once created it continues forever. These words can be imagined floating into the Universe where it will be fine-tuned by the guides and sent back in a form not yet realized by the sender. Know that it is released and being nurtured, because that is the key to success. When anything is held tightly to the physical it can suffocate and die.

*If you love it, set it free.*
*If it comes back, it is yours.*
*If it does not, it never was.*

An age old phrase, but so true. Not only do we need to let go of ideals and concepts, but we must let go of how we hold on to the way people should be as well. The release will bring back more in return. We are the creators of our reality and we have the ability to manifest the life we desire. As one works in tandem with the powers of the Universe, together great things can be accomplished. If an idea is held to only be valuable in one form, there is no space for the Universe to create something better. Make the request, let it go, trust that it will be fulfilled and offer thanks for its fulfillment.

Days or weeks later, check in on your desire which is held in a bubble. If the image appears different, ask the all knowing presence of your higher self why. Perhaps the color or intensity has changed. The changing of color may be showing you what chakra is being adjusted to receive your gift. If it looks foggy you may need to wait for clarity to arise from a situation. Bring the vision closer if that feels appropriate or allow it to have distance. It may be moving away to give you a new perspective or to connect to another person who will assist in manifesting your desire. There is information in this bubble; be still and listen. Each time you visit your request, tune into the feeling of receiving the gift. Notice the sensations in your body, emotions and thoughts. Make the necessary changes and remember it is the feelings that power your affirmation.

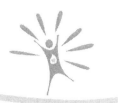

**Example:** My desire for years was to bring in a loving partner. The day before he walked into my life I asked my friend Sandra if she would conduct a hypnosis session with me. The reason for the session was to inquire as to why Bob, my high school sweetheart, was coming up to Denver for a visit. Bob and I had remained friends over 40 years and have communicated on occasion but this visit had me puzzled. He claimed his tour was his desire to ride his motorcycle from Tucson to Denver and enjoy the mountains in celebration of his 60th birthday. It seemed plausible to me but this event still had me curious.

Sandra, who is a very good hypno-therapist, sat down with me and conducted a hypnosis session. For we knew, the answer was within my subconscious mind...the part that knows and can reveal all. A Reiki session will bring one into the subconscious state as well and that is why Reiki is so efficient in revealing old issues.

Not long into our session, I could feel love all around me; it was so close I could touch it. I knew this was the soft, loving light of my divine partner and he was very near. Sandra could feel it as well. It was so beautiful we both were touched by emotion but I never thought this was a reflection of Bob. What came to be the next day was the arrival of my old friend and a rekindling of our love. I am blessed to say we are now married and living our dream.

The love Sandra and I felt is the energy I am referring to. When a desire is sent out and allowed to develop, it draws to it what is needed for its manifestation. I did not need to bring my desire any closer to me; I could feel it and I knew at that time my divine partner was near. I was not given the information that it was Bob for that would have lessened the joy of finding our love, in the moment. I knew love was close at last and I relaxed. Once Bob and I again met and opened our hearts to each other, it was so comforting to find the relationship I was waiting for was someone whom I have known and loved since I was 15.

Do not try to push your image out into the Universe telling it how things "should be". The Universe, as I found out, will supply you with more than you could have possibility imagined. So let go and trust all will be given in divine order.

## Releasing Addictions

Sei-He-Ki can assist in removing addictions because it will not only work with present time struggles but goes into the past to uncover the core issue. When the original issue is understood and compassionately released the subsequent issues will also drop away. Reiki brings the problems to the surface where the recipients may better understand why they have made their current choices.

 **Remember:** Do not infringe on another's free-will choice.
Stay unattached to the results.

Reiki works 100% of the time, but the process may not always be physically evident. Reiki flows through and adjusts the physical, mental, emotional and spiritual bodies. With your assistance, the recipient can become aware of which body is being adjusted. In the case of addictions, this habit becomes a way to hide emotional and physical pain. These old issues must be addressed before one will be able to release the addiction. Sei-He-Ki gently brings these memories to the surface. Reiki is always guided by the higher self of the recipient; therefore the highest essence of the client is in control of what is presented. Reiki never brings to the surface any more than the recipient can handle at any given time. If they are made aware of an old issue, they are ready to work with and clear it. The practitioner acts as the support while the client moves through their issues at their own pace.

Often family members want to help a loved one afflicted with an addictive behavior. They will ask you to send Reiki to that one, but make sure you or the family member does not have an expectation for the outcome. The subject has free will and Reiki enters with the guidance by their higher self. In some cases, the

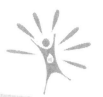

Reiki can be blocked if they are not ready to let go of the cause of the addiction. Reiki will stay with them in a bubble of light until they are open to receive the positive support of Reiki. Even if it takes years or a life time, the love of Reiki will stay with them indefinitely; this love will travel with them and bless them even when they are on the other side after death. Reiki always works and it will bless them with love and light; no gift given is ever wasted. If the addiction still is prevalent, know that Reiki is blessing their form in the way they can receive at this time.

Addictions for the most part have an anchor in the throat chakra. If you think about it, all addictive substances enter this chakra: liquor, drugs, excess food, smoke, even harsh words. When working with an addictive personality, spend some time directing Reiki with Sei-He-Ki to the throat chakra. Then proceed to other parts of the body as you are guided.

Uncovering the Underlying Cause

The mental and emotional symbol allows healing to occur at a deeper level, at the root of the cause. The body is a messenger, sending out pain and various ailments in order to get a person's attention. It directs one to look deeper within for answers.

Pain may first be felt in the physical body but the core issues are held in the emotional, mental or spiritual bodies. If they are not addressed, they will manifest into the physical body, where they cannot be ignored. Meditation and focusing within the body can assist in locating the issues that are creating the physical problems. Information can be found if one attunes to the body's needs. In our society we are taught to ignore the body and mask the symptoms. Reiki will give the eager student access to pertinent information thus allowing self-healing to begin.

Listen to how the body is relating information. What is it saying? What is the direction it is pointing to? Is it revealing doorways where emotions can be transcended? Movement towards an answer will only occur when the underlying issues are found. View these issues as experiences rather than criticism. Don't judge them as good or bad, see them only as information.

Help the client to acknowledge their part in creating the struggle and make a different choice. The mental and emotional symbol helps to give the power to do just that. It opens the doors into the psyche that need to be aired out and revealed. Do not fear that the information will take the client into overload. If an issue arises, then on some level they are ready to look at it and work through it.

*~Life does not give us any more that we can handle~*

## Eating Disorders, Self Image & Smoking

Sei-He-Ki can be used to release unwanted habits because it works within the mental and emotional parameters so it can alleviate the underlying cause of the negative tendency. When unwanted habits stay stuck in the energy field the heart requires attention. The lack of self love is prevalent either consciously or unconsciously. The entire healing process is supported by the love Reiki channels into the client.

## Weight Balancing

If someone wants to change their weight, write the name of the person who wants to adjust their size on a piece of paper along with the positive way to approach this habit. One statement could be balanced healthy eating or eating

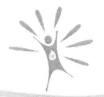

only when the body requires nourishment. To give the client support to manifest their desire, daily direct Reiki into the paper, which holds their desire.

The best way to change eating patterns is to discover when and why one eats in an unhealthy way. Ask yourself or the client, am I really hungry or is eating at this time an emotional act? The reason could be not only habit, but stress, loneliness or feelings of unworthiness. It may be the lack of knowledge about the proper diet for their personal body and blood type, which can trip up the most adamant dieter.

Many Americans have no idea what foods are good for their individual body. There is no need to be an expert in every subject, but it does aid the client if you know where to send them for more information. You can be a resource directory, rather than an encyclopedia. Most people eat too many carbohydrates and this excess can create cravings which are often fed by Candida. Candida is an over abundance of yeast in the body which is aggravated by eating starch, sugar and alcohol.

A few books on the subject of what our particular body may need are: *Eat Right for your Type, by* Dr. Peter D'Adamo and *Dr. Abravanel's Body Type Diet and Lifetime Nutrition Plan* by Dr. Elliot Abravanel and Elizabeth A. King. To stop craving carbohydrates, *The Carbohydrate Addict's Lifespan Program* by Heller is a good choice. These books are some examples to get you started but when it comes to dieting there is a myriad of data at your disposal. Directing clients to books pertinent to their needs can be very helpful.

Everyone is unique and there are numerous reasons why weight is held on the body. Those differences comprise how each person can eat healthy. The process is not the same for all but there are models to follow.

## Self-Image

When there is a weight problem, the best course of action is to look at how the client defines their self image. More than likely this area of their life needs tweaking. After confidence and self love is built with Reiki treatments, diet and exercise programs may be incorporated. Until then, one is only wasting their time and frustrating the client. The body is a shell for the emotions and reflects what is held therein. Release the judgment, guilt and sadness before attempting weight control. Hands-on healing focuses on opening the heart, which will increase the success rate of any weight changing program. Once the heart is light, the body will want to begin to move and the simple act of walking can be a good start.

When the body is out of balance, often that person is depressed and has no motivation to do much of anything, let alone start a weight loss program. In an effort to mask their emotions, they will check out by watching television and often sleep excessively. In this way they do not face or feel their pain. When one feels good about themselves they will not eat because of stress or depression and it will feel good to move their body and therefore exercise. The support received from a Reiki treatment will direct universal light into the body, which is love. This will build a foundation for continued wellness; physically, mentally and emotionally.

## Smoking

Smoking addictions are similar to weight balancing in that it could come from depression and stress. Smoking is a way to remove yourself from a situation, make a statement of independence, slow down your energy and, for some, relax. But it is also a statement of "I do not want to be in this body." With all the information at our disposal about the dangers of smoking, it is hard to believe the person who smokes has a strong desire to live. When you find the underlying cause of the destructive behavior and heal it with Reiki, the destructive habit will dissolve. The

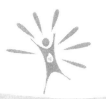

most challenging part of this treatment is finding a client who truly wants to stop this habit. I have seen many people say they want to quit but deep within this is not their heart's desire.

For cigarette addiction, work with the client to help them discover why they smoke and what makes it enjoyable for them. Some people smoke in order to have an excuse to take a break. In many offices, there are no longer the common coffee breaks of the past, now employees are expected to work through the day without a reprieve. But when it comes to smokers, they are given the time to walk away from work and converge with fellow employees who indulge in the same habit. Along with this break comes the whole social aspect of smoking. For these reasons alone, smokers could be holding onto their addiction.

**Example:** I have found when I ask a smoker why they smoke, many of them say they enjoy that first long, slow, deep breath. My thought is why not slow down from life and take that relaxing deep breath without the cigarette. So for these clients I introduce them to breathing techniques which allow them to relax for a moment, bring in oxygen and deep breath without smoke going down into their lungs. I suggest they try following their usual pattern of taking a pause but don't light up. When they are ready for their cigarette break, step out into the fresh air and take a few long slow deep breaths. They could find this aspect alone will help ease the desire to smoke.

While supporting a client in the wish to stop smoking, help them find a positive affirmation for their inner focus. Once the affirmation is constructed, have the client physically write it on a paper so it holds their fingerprint. Remind them to look at the paper during the day as a reminder that a new habit is being formed.

 **Remember:** Create a statement which reflects
gratitude in the future tense.

If the affirmation states, "I am smoke free," it highlights the old pattern and could reactivate the old habit. Make the statement an affirmation of the reflection of your fulfilled desire, such as, "I love how my lungs always fill with fresh clean air." Hold the focus on what is desired, not what is being released.

 Life Tool: Deep Breathing Technique to Stop Smoking

| |
|---|
| 1. Breathe in through your mouth for the count of four. |
| 2. Breathe out through your mouth for the count of eight. |
| 3. As lung capacity increases, raise the number of the count, always doubling the number on the exhale as compared to the inhale. |
| 4. Physically raise the lower abdomen as your body fills with air. Expand the chest as the rib cage spreads as you continue to inhale. |
| 5. On the exhale, release the air first from the chest and then contract the stomach muscles as the stomach moves back towards the spine as the old air is pushed out. |
| 6. The exercise begins with the breath into the mouth to mimic the sensation of smoking. |
| 7. After a few weeks, switch breathing through the mouth to breathing through the nose. |
| 8. Remind client before they reach for a cigarette to stop and breathe in this fashion for 10 breaths. The craving for a cigarette just could subside or at least greatly lessen. |

## Spirit Attachments

Often when a habit persists, the addicted person is not only dealing with their own addiction, but with other unseen energies as well. These covert forms are what make releasing an addiction so complex. When people pass on, even though

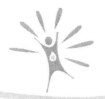

their body is gone, they do not always leave the earth. The spirit sometimes lingers. They stay when they feel there is unfinished business or when they have a strong addictive behavior.

For clients who would question this type of thinking, it can be explained in this less radical manner. Everything on the earth has an electrical energy and a vibrational movement. Addictive behavior magnetically draws to itself behavior of a like kind. Smokers know this for a fact; they almost inherently recognize each other in a group. In the work place they will meet at the location which is designated for smoking and become comrades. This common bond is not only physical; it is magnetic, thus energetic. Then it becomes a difficult connection to break, but it can be made easier with the imagery of cutting the cords which bind them together.

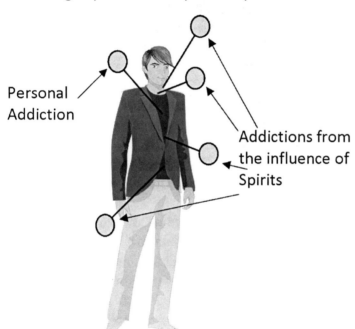

Personal Addiction

Addictions from the influence of Spirits

We are comprised of energy and energy cannot be destroyed; it can be changed, but it will always exist. When an individual passes out of the body in death, the energy preferably will ascend to a higher dimension. However, not all spirits leave this earthly plane immediately. Some stay in the earthly realm to enjoy the pleasures of the flesh. These spirits will desire to be close to those who are in a body and who are addicted to the same substance the spirit craved when it was in a body. Their presence can increase addictive desires in a human being. The person with the addiction is not possessed, they just require the energy field around them to be cleared of these forces.

## Why Entities Stay

If a spirit has not moved on after passing, there are reasons for their connection to the earth. Often, when the motive is discovered, you have the ability to release the entity. Movies have depicted how these strange scenarios might occur. Films are not just fantasies; often they hold a semblance of truth. The story in *The Sixth Sense* portrays a small boy who is haunted by a ghost who appears to be only interested in scaring him. The boy hides in a tent and peeks outside, finding the young spirit vomiting. But fear is not what drove her to connect with this boy. She wanted him to help her sister. When this girl was alive, she had been poisoned by her mentally ill mother. Because of her stressful death she carried the affliction which killed her into the other side. She did not want to scare the boy; she was only in search of his help. She wanted the boy to save her sister's life because her sister was now being poisoned by her mother as well.

When it comes to addictions, the spirits are released when they are recognized and asked to leave. If the entity does not leave, use the guided imagery of the "Life Tool, Releasing Spirit Attachments." This will reveal the deeper reasons for their continued presence. Once the information is uncovered the client has the wisdom and power to stand as master of their personal space and say who is welcome within it. Once the information is received as to why the disembodied being is there, they may quickly disappear. If not, the client or host needs to command strongly that this entity's presence is no longer desired and it must leave.

When more assistance is required, know there are constructive spirit beings whose only purpose is to help those lost out of body souls onto their next level. The problem occurs when a soul thinks it still has a physical form and is alive. Because of this confusion their attention is directed only to people in human form

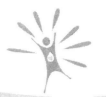

and they do not recognize the angels, guides and helpers who are on the other side trying to help them. They only imagine conversing with humans on earth. The main character in *The Sixth Sense* was so assured he was still in human form, he convinced the audience of this also. I think that it took most people until the end of the movie to see he too was a spirit confused about where he belonged.

If we want to assist the spirit who has passed on, we do not need to know where they need to go or how. Introducing the spirit to the divine helpers on the other side is all that is required, nothing more. The helper will take it from there. There is no need to be concerned that this process is too advanced for you, for the helper is doing all the work, you only make their acquaintance.

Stay with the imagery and observe what happens next. Keep your intuition activated as it can be very interesting to watch. But, remember you do not need to participate in the removal of the soul. It will be taken care of by the divine light beings. Once your client's energy field is clear, continue to support them with the Reiki symbols and a Reiki treatment, but ultimately it will be up to your client to call their power back. The love of Reiki will empower and support this activity.

Other Entity Forms

Negative habits and unhealthy behavior over time will take on a life of their own. They will build in intensity until they become an energetic entity. Every time a person becomes angry and out of control, as in the case of anger or road rage, a negative thought form is created. It builds in power every time a harsh word is expressed. Over time this thought form will grow in power until it becomes so strong it forms an entity which needs to be dissolved and released. These are not disembodied beings or ghosts. They are self created mental forms that have become so strong they take on the qualities of entities. They will try to take control of a person's life and often succeed. They can be difficult to rid from the energy field because they were created by the very one who is trying to release this destructive tendency. Once the client is made consciously aware of their creation they can release it quickly by merely creating an alternate desire, this will disband it.

Whether it is an entity which once had form in a body or an entity created by strong vicious thoughts, they will both be removed with the following "Life Tool." Begin to open the client toward becoming aware of unseen energies by asking them to visualize the images as you guide them.

 **Remember:** Prime the pump of the inner sight of your client with the guided imagery of the appropriate "Life Tool."

The process of using imagery will assist and open the client to become aware of unseen activities in their body and aura. Inform them that even if they do not see or sense what you are saying, pretend that they do. In this way, they are tricking the left brain into thinking the process is actually happening. The definition of pretend is to play, or to make up, so guide the client to pretend their crown chakra is opening and a light is flowing in. To activate the right brain we want to stimulate the senses by requesting the recipient imagine a color along with a temperature. Let them follow the flow of light down into each and every chakra sharing a color and temperature along the way. Usually by the time they arrive at the solar plexus and often the heart they will comment that they are actually feeling a sensation. Now the client is open to see with their inner sight and uncover the needed information to successfully complete the process.

 **Remember:** A client can always make up what they do not see or sense.

Ask that they bring in an angel and have it stand on their right side. They will be aware of their presence by a temperature change, a light physical touch or just by knowing it. Now invite a guide who can lead the process they are about to enter. Color is the simplest thing to perceive in the mind, so start with that question. Ask them to notice the color of each of these beings as well as their size, brightness and intensity.

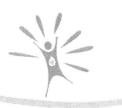

Next introduce the client to their own divine essence. What is the size, is it larger or smaller than their guide or angel? The client is often surprised to find their divine self is as large and bright as the guides and angels they have called in for assistance. This becomes a very empowering visualization. If their higher self is smaller or less bright than the guide or angel, instruct the client to turn up their light just like turning up the lights with a dimmer on the wall. Now their confidence and power is intensified and they are ready to start.

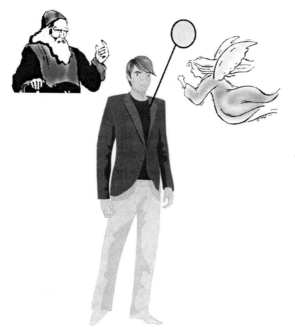

Assistance from guide & angel to release spirits

If communication with the spirit becomes strained or nonexistent at any time during the process, use the following technique. Asking yes and no questions, tell the spirit to bounce up and down for a yes response and back and forth for no. This will soon get the information flowing.

The cutting of energy lines from a person to a spirit will make them feel lighter as they are no longer carrying the afflictions of this out of body being. This will also empower the client, for now, they will not have the outside influence of another. When calling in help from divine beings, the Reiki practitioner can often sense the power of these ascended forms even if they do not know exactly who they are. A practitioner will sense they are not alone as they work with the removal of a force which cannot be seen.

When the practitioner directs the client to call for the assistance of a divine being or sacred fire image, such as the Sword of Archangel Michael it can give a

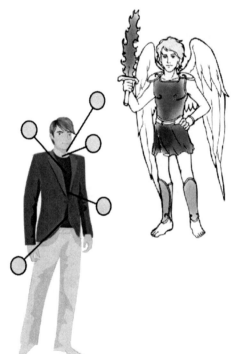

sense of power over their addiction. They have now given the esoteric a form and they have an image to hold on to. This gives them the strength to wield force over the addiction which is also unseen and has been haunting them and draining their energy. Instruct the client how to use the Sword of Blue Flame to cut themselves free from the lines of force which hold them to their addiction. Through guided imagery introduce them to Archangel Michael or a divine being of their choosing.

Disembodied beings, entities or energy attachments can be released by using Sei-He-Ki and calling in the assistance of powerful angels such as Archangel Michael. Sei-He-Ki brings emotional issues to the surface while Archangel Michael cuts the

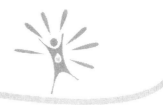

individual free from the attachment to the cause.

Sei-He-Ki will be used along with Cho-Ku-Rei and the distant symbol. Then Reiki will be enhanced with the use of these symbols. Cho-Ku-Rei will increase the power needed on all levels. Sei-He-Ki will insure the original core issue will be understood and brought to the surface for clearing. The distant symbol, presented in Chapter 4, will touch and clear all time frames: past, present and future.

Archangel Michael is a cosmic being who is known throughout many religious communities. He wields a sword of power and love which on the esoteric level, appears to have blue flames emanating from its blade. By the use of this sword the holder will feel its support as it has the ability to cut the user free from anything that binds or limits them.

## Using Archangel Michael to release spirits

When there is an addiction such as smoking, liquor, drugs, anger or food, there is often an entity which has attached itself to the person who is addicted. The entity draws on the energy of the individual, creating the yearning for the addiction even when the person has a strong desire to stop their unhealthy life style. When attempting to alleviate an old habit, one might feel as if they have no control over their own body and in a sense they do not. The entity is adding to the uncontrollable desires within and the habitual sensations.

The Sword of Blue Flame could be visualized as a beautiful sword with jewels on the hilt and blue flames shooting out of the blade. The recipient or the practitioner may imagine a different picture. There is no wrong way to perceive the sword and adding a personal touch is always acceptable as the information here given are only suggestions. Let your imagination or that of the client take command; then it becomes their process and it empowers them as the user.

Reach up and take hold of the sword and sever all attachment lines from the client to the entity forms. If appropriate, show the client how to cut the lines also. Request that the client create a visual form of a sword which reflects power in their minds eye. Ask Archangel Michael to place his hand over theirs as they reach up and take hold of it. They will then bring down the sword and cut all attachments around their body. Show the client how they can use this transcendent sword to cut themselves free anytime they feel the desire for the old addictions.

The use of Archangel Michael's Sword of Blue Flame can cut one free from numerous entities held in the aura. These spirits are attached by cords which are hooked into the human form. The beauty of using this sword is that not only does it cut one free but it does it in love, as the flame sears and seals the cords so that there are no frayed edges. If raw edges were left untouched, there could be an irritation lingering in the emotional body.

Once the decision is made to release an addiction, it will take 21 days to create a new habit. Continually cutting attachments during the 21-day integration period will assist in the release of the addiction. Remind the client to cut the unseen addictions throughout the day.

**Example:** Many cigarette smokers have an intense desire for a cigarette just after a meal. If they apply the above process to cut the lines of attachment as they prepare their meal the desire for a cigarette will be lessened after the meal.

 Life Tool: Releasing Spirit Attachments

> 1. Have recipient lie on a massage table and begin a hands-on healing treatment to open to the subconscious mind, the place where change permanently occurs.

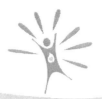

| |
|---|
| 2. Verbally guide them through the opening of their chakras, instruct them as follows. |
|    a.   Imagine an iridescent light entering the top of your head. |
|    b.  Iridescent light contains all colors: what color do you imagine? If no color comes to mind, make one up. |
|    c.  What is the temperature? Again pretend it is warm or cool if no sensation is felt. |
|    d.  With your mind's eye, let the light flow into your forehead. This is the third eye and it activates a light beam in the all-seeing eye of your intuition. The color may change to blue. Is it cool or warm? |
|    e.  The light continues to open the heart chakra in the chest cavity. As the heart opens pretend you can breathe deeper as your chest broadens to accommodate the expansion. |
|    f.  Keep the energy moving as it drops into the stomach, this is the solar plexus and it houses the emotions. The color is yellow, are you feeling any calmer as the light fills this center? |
|    g.  As the light moves lower in the body it will enter the sacral chakra, the color is orange and it embodies our creative essence. |
|    h.  The last chakra resides at the bottom of the spine; it is the base chakra and connects us to the earth. This grounding activity helps keep us in present time and can relieve stress. Imagine a breeze entering as it opens. |
| 3. Ask for a guide to appear and join in the process. |
|    a.  The guide is one who has knowledge about the spirit that will be released and will lead the process. |
|    b.  Place the guide on your left side. |
|    c.  Let me know when you are aware of their presence by a touch, temperature or inner knowing. |
| 4. Request for an angel to enter and have them stand at your right |

| |
|---|
| shoulder. |
|    a.  The angel is here to give love and protection. |
|    b.  Let me know when you are aware of their presence |
| 5. Look at your body on the table and step back so you may observe the essence of your higher self. |
|    a.  What is the color, intensity and size of your higher spirit? |
|    b.  Compare the illumination of your higher self to that of the guide and angel. |
|    c.  If they are not equal then bring up your illumination by turning up a light switch. |
| 6. Place the spirit to be released in front of you. |
| 7. Begin a conversation with the spirit. Some questions could be: |
|    a.  Why are you here with me? |
|    b.  Do you want to tell me something? |
|    c.  What do you want from me? |
|    d.  How may I help you move on? |
| 8. If there are difficulties communicating, merely ask the spirit to answer by bouncing up and down for a yes response and moving back and forth for no. |
| 9. Depending on the answers, the spirit may leave on its own or stay, requesting further assistance. If support is required, call in a helper. |
| 10.    Your job is to introduce the spirit to the helper, nothing more. The helper will take it from there. |
| 11.    If desired, you and the client may watch and see where the helper is taking the spirit. |
| 12.    Complete the process with a full hands-on healing treatment. |

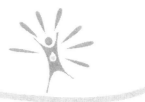

Why does the release become permanent?

A problem or cord can be released permanently when the core issue is found and cleared. This is done in present time but is addressed in the past time when it occurred. When these time frames are traversed, the scenario is rewritten and body systems can readjust. It is as if the incident never happened.

Time is an illusion; it is created by our linear left mind. It allows us the ability to conceptualize the vastness of the universe we live in and beyond. Our minds imagine a line of time and thought but actually all time occurs simultaneously. Without this time continuum our thoughts, or electrical circuits, become overloaded, causing electrical short circuiting.

The time levels we can access are past, present, future and parallel. Past, present and future are part of our linear timeline but parallel time frames bring in another part of conceptual time. Parallel realities are intervals which happen simultaneously with present time. Every decision we make has a counter decision that we did not make. For instance, in present time you are reading this book, but in a parallel period of time you made an alternate decision and that aspect of self is off doing another activity. These other time frames sometimes become enmeshed with present time and that is when the problem occurs.

Using of the distant symbol will make sure all levels of reality are cleared so the attachment will not connect again. This symbol will be taught in the next chapter.

Understanding and Intuiting New Perceptions

The mental and emotional well-being of a client can be enhanced by directing Sei-He-Ki into their bodies: physical, mental, emotional and spiritual. Reiki is guided by the higher self and therefore will uncover what is holding the person back. As a practitioner you may receive personal guidance about the situation before the client does; hold back this information. Always honor the client's ability to perceive their own guidance because under the umbrella of Reiki their intuition will increase. What they discover themselves will have more worth than what you will give them, but your intuitive insights are also valuable. Filter in your information at the appropriate time or keep it to yourself if the opportunity does not present itself. Sometimes the information you intuitively receive is to help you proceed in the treatment and was never meant to be shared.

Ask for direction from their highest source and follow the instruction given. In this way, the true cause of the issues of the addiction or dis-ease in the body will surface in the way that is best for them. When the individual is not balanced, the body becomes uneasy with its current predicament, hence the term dis-ease.

It's funny but people usually comprehend what they are being told if they see it in print. So back up your intuitive guidance with published facts. When you have a hit as to why the client is in their present dilemma direct them to one of the following books. The ones I return to again and again list ailments and emotions often reflected from various diseases. *Heal your Body* by Louise Hays is a quick reference book that is compact, inexpensive and easy to carry. More comprehensive and detailed is *Feelings Buried Alive Never Die* by Karol Truman. The list of ailments is extensive with as many as 15 emotions tied to a dis-ease. It is surprising how often it ties in with just the situations which have been occurring in the client's life, both present and past. The client often sees this confirmation as an "aha," as to an emotion which has been buried.

Because so many people are unaware of how emotions affect their body, these books shine a light on places which have been held in the shadows. Once brought to conscious awareness, the problem has arisen and can no longer hold the recipient at bay. Now illumined on their path, the client can move forward. Just the simple act of revealing the connection to old incidents can start the process for an immense healing.

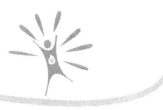

# Chapter 4


## The Distant Symbol

---

The distant symbol allows us to access information and address issues in alternate time frames and remote locations. Because Reiki is merely energy, it can travel at the speed of thought through time or miles and the protocol used is the same for time or distance. There is no limit to where Reiki healing can go or how it can serve us or others.

Now whenever a Reiki treatment is begun, all three Reiki symbols will be used. Cho-Ku-Rei will seal the space in love and activate the power of Reiki. Sei-He-Ki will make sure the emotional issues will surface with compassion and mental clarity. The distant symbol, Hon-Sha-Ze-Sho-Nen, will direct the healing light to the core issue in any time frame or move the energy across the miles if the client is not physically present.

## Hon-Sha-Ze-Sho-Nen, the Distant Symbol

Pronunciation: (Hon Sha Zay Show Nin)

Translation:

Hon:
> center
> essence
> origin or start
> intrinsic (it is already there)

Sha:
> shimmering

Ze:
> advancing correct course

Sho or Shyo:
> target       integrity
> honest man     honest being
>  a sage  (a wise man)

Nen:
> stillness
> thinking by keeping in the deepest
>    part of the mind

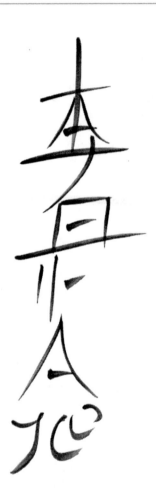

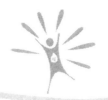

Memory is enhanced by colors, therefore, to remember this symbol draw each section in a different color. Each syllable is a section. Draw the numbers in the corresponding sections in different colors as well. This will become an imprint in the mind and aid in memorizing this form.

.

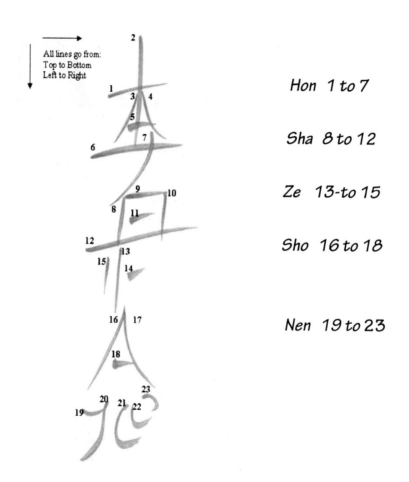

All lines go from:
Top to Bottom
Left to Right

Hon  1 to 7

Sha  8 to 12

Ze  13-to 15

Sho  16 to 18

Nen  19 to 23

Hon-Sha-Ze-Sho-Nen is used to direct the healing of Reiki across the miles and also through the dimension of time: past, present or future. Like using hands-on healing, the intent becomes the strongest attribute. Ask for the healing to be given to another and it is granted. Sending Reiki at a distance is not as esoteric as one might think. Reiki is like prayer: it can travel as fast as thought.

Prove to yourself how fast thought travels and how the visual mind responds. Begin by thinking about the Statue of Liberty in New York City. What comes to mind: the water, the torch, her crown? In a sense, you were just there. That is how fast energy moves and it is done with the least amount of effort, purely with thought. There is a protocol for dispersing Reiki through time and space which you will see shortly. Following this method will bring healing, which often can be even stronger than direct hands-on healing. In actuality, Reiki will begin to flow the moment the client places their request.

*~ The call compels the answer ~*

The act of asking opens a channel of light from the client's higher self so they may receive the energy. The healing comes from the same source, whether it is channeled from the Reiki practitioner to the recipient or if the recipient asks Source directly. The energy is flowing from the Universe through a grid that connects us to the oneness which flows through all life. This grid was seen and drawn by the artist Alex Grey, his images can be viewed in his book *Sacred Mirrors.*

Reiki can never be used for harm, nor can it carry any negativity. Any of the processes given in this book cannot be preformed incorrectly. If the intent is to assist another, the request shall be granted. When Reiki is added to the mix, love flows and all is placed in divine order. So do not fret, you do not have to follow

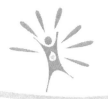

this manual as it is exactly stated. Allow your intuition to direct you; this book carries guidelines, that is all.

There is no wrong way to pray, nor is there a wrong way to send Reiki. Reiki is pure love; there is no way to share this energy incorrectly. As with prayer, when a request for healing is made, it immediately goes out to the recipient without question. The answer to a prayer is given as soon as it is sent; it is human doubt which blocks the receiver from accessing the reply. With Reiki, the healing also happens instantaneously, but may go unnoticed when the results lie in the etheric bodies.

 **Remember:** Reiki works on all four bodies: physical, mental, emotional and spiritual. The results can go unseen if the client is not made aware of where to look.

Healing occurs through the opening of the heart and the connection to the love, which emanates from every living thing on earth. Healing love is in the beauty of the sunset, the smell of rain, the awe of infinity, which in turn integrates into Reiki. Because the basis of Reiki is love, it has the ability to open the recipient's heart with transcendent love sent through universal life force energy and the practitioners' hands. Reiki connects to this love and channels it into the bodies.

Moving beyond dis-ease can come through medical treatment, medicinal drugs, herbs, alternative care or sheer will.

*~ Love is the ultimate healer ~*

There is a point when the patient will make a decision to open, receive and accept the love they deserve and this allows the healing to begin. Reiki supports this decision. A Reiki treatment can begin even before a client arrives by sending distant healing to a client before their appointment, thus allowing them to relax and be more receptive to the session. A simple and quick way to achieve this is to send Reiki into your daily appointments the previous evening.

Healing at a Distance

Distant Reiki works like hands-on Reiki. When it is received by the recipient, their higher self directs the energy into the part of the body where it will be of most value. The term "sending Reiki" is often used, but it is actually not sent, it is drawn. When a treatment begins the crown of the practitioner is opened, the energy flows into their heart, out their hands and into the client. The client's higher self then directs the energy to where it is required. The practitioner might notice energy being drawn out of their hands as the higher self of the client imparts the healing light. It could be directed into the physical, mental, emotional or spiritual body. The practitioner opens to the universal life force energy of Reiki and with clear intent asks for it to be directed to the recipient.

 **Remember:** We as healers are the channels through which the energy flows. Keep this in mind when the term "send" is used.

All three symbols are used before a Reiki second degree healing treatment. When beginning a treatment, start with Cho-Ku-Rei to convey power and protection. This will open to the supremacy of Reiki and seal the energy of those involved. Then the practitioner will not take on the struggles of the recipient and the recipient will not be affected by any issues the practitioner may have that day.

Next, draw Sei-He-Ki to bring to the surface new perceptions for any mental and emotional problems. Know that only the issues which the client is ready to face will surface, along with an appropriate solution. Using Hon-Sha-Ze-Sho-Nen will direct the magnitude of Reiki to the correct time frame, past, present or future and across the miles as necessary. Any time during the treatment the symbols can be used individually, but the power lies in the use of all three together at the start of the treatment. As always, Cho-Ku-Rei will be drawn at the

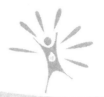

end of the treatment to anchor the client back into their body and to place their healing into the earth as well as their physical form.

With Hon-Sha-Ze-Sho-Nen, Reiki can be transmitted across a room, a town, or a country. Therefore the Reiki practitioner does not need to be physically present with the client for the energy to be received. Often distant healing can be felt stronger than when a hands-on treatment is given.

The distant symbol is only a vehicle to carry the healing force. Hon-Sha-Ze-Sho-Nen directs the healing to the dimension where the issue originated. Time is only an illusion of three dimensional reality. The love found in Reiki moves beyond time and space, into the place where the deepest healing can occur. It can move into past events, past lives, future happenings or a future existence. There is no limit to where it can be sent or how it can be received.

The symbols are drawn in the air and their names are spoken out loud if no one else is in the room, otherwise their names are chanted silently. This is done not because the symbols are secret; it is done because they are sacred. Once the symbol is activated, a connection is made to anyone who has ever used these symbols by the vibration which is created by drawing and speaking the names of the symbols. A correlation is created, bringing in not only the power of your higher self, but also healing assistance from all that have used the symbols in the past. This is a very powerful realization.

The Reiki second-degree attunement embeds the symbols into the subconscious mind. The drawing and the speaking of the symbols eventually create a pattern from which the practitioner receives higher energy. Over time they will find the energy of the symbols will be there for their use even when the symbols have not been drawn. The time it takes for this to happen is up to the Reiki student. It may be months or years, but it will happen. The power of Reiki is beyond the conscious mind. As the apprentice lets go and moves into the flow of Reiki, all of their healing abilities will be at their call as quick as a thought.

Reiki always works 100% of the time, but the results may not be seen at first in the physical body. When the physical ailment does not immediately disappear, it is not reflecting the inability of Reiki to heal, it is just telling you to look at another place. Reiki moves through all levels of consciousness: physical, mental, emotional and spiritual. When the physical ailment persists, the energy could be clearing the spiritual body. This may be seen as an appreciation for nature or an opening to self-love by a gentle release of self judgment. Within the emotional body, kind reminders may be present to assure the recipient that all is in divine order and that what has been emotionally upsetting in the past is a gift in disguise. The gift will be revealed by their divine self along with a clear understanding of how this is happening. The mental body could heal with the sheer fact that it becomes calm and ideas are activated and clear. Many clients feel stress being released during a treatment which is the clearing within their mental body.

## Distant Healing Protocol

There is an order to follow when giving Reiki over the miles, but your intuitive nature may alter this line up, therefore change it at your discretion. Begin by drawing the three basic Reiki symbols:

❖ *Cho-Ku-Rei* will amplify the healing energy as well as seal the space in light around the giver and the receiver.
❖ *Sei-He-Ki* mentally and emotionally clarifies the issue while opening the client to new perceptions.
❖ *Hon-Sha-Ze-Sho-Nen* sends the healing light across the miles and into all time frames and dimensions.

Stating the name of the recipient assures the healing will be going to the correct address so to speak. The quantity of three holds the energy of the trinity, so the name is repeated three times honoring the sacredness of this number. Hold the reflection of the client in your mind and if you have never met, just pretend to see them. Make up a visual form, the intent to help holds the power, not the

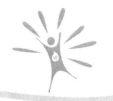

perfection of the image. Inquire as to the age, physical qualities, approximate place they reside, the hospital where they are a patient and any other information they wish to share. When the healing intent is directed to the recipient their heart opens to accept the energy flowing in, as does the heart of the practitioner.

 **Remember:** When Reiki is given, it is directed by the higher self of the recipient releasing the practitioner of responsibility for the results.

When the practitioner asks for Reiki to flow, it first comes into their own chakras and then out to another where their higher self will take over and direct it into the appropriate bodies. This relieves the giver of responsibility as to how it heals, for it is divinely guided. You may have your palms facing away from you as you direct the energy through your hands to the recipient. There could be a building of energy in your palms or the sense of energy being drawn from your hands as it moves out to the client. Another way is to imagine the client in between your hands as you direct Reiki into them. You may feel more energy in one part of your hands which reflects a particular part of their body. If so, find out if they have had a problem at any time in this area to confirm your intuition.

The treatment can last up to 20 minutes but the energy may feel like it shuts off after as little as five minutes. This is a signal the session is complete, but as you close the treatment, request that the energy continues to flow as long as they need it. Draw the three Reiki symbols and release the client by your intent to do so. This is accomplished by blowing on your hands as if you are gently propelling them home, visually release their energy to the earth or in a manner of your choice. Do what feels right to you and remember the basic premise of Reiki is the clients do not take on your energy and you do not take on theirs, even after the treatment. If you do feel you have harbored some of their problems, it can be because they are mirroring back to you an issue you have held in your own field. Refer to one of the books on emotions and how they effect the body to see where your similarities lie and then just ask them to clear. Releasing old issues can be as easy as making that clear intent.

Life Tool:  Healing at a Distance

| | |
|---|---|
| 1. | Draw the power symbol, Cho-Ku-Rei and chant the name. |
| 2. | Draw the mental/emotional symbol, Sei-He-Ki and say the name. |
| 3. | Draw the distant symbol, Hon-Sha-Ze-Sho-Nen and repeat its name. |
| 4. | Voice the recipient's name three times. |
| 5. | Visualize that person as best you can. |
| 6. | Connect heart to heart. |
| 7. | Hold your hands out, direct Reiki to them and notice any sensations in your hands or body. |
| 8. | Time needed is up to 20 minutes or until the energy subsides. |
| 9. | Release the client energetically with intent. |
| 10. | Close by drawing all three symbols again, ending with Cho-Ku-Rei to seal in the healing light. |

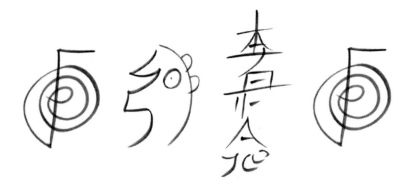

Order of how symbols are drawn before a treatment

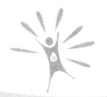

The focus does not always need to be on the recipient while transmitting Reiki: Reiki will flow even if the attention of the practitioner is not on the healing process. Once the intent is made to give Reiki, the light begins to flow, but paying attention to the sensations holds a value. By staying attentive to the energy, information will arise to help with the healing process. Feel the energy; let it merge with you as it flows through you because when you give Reiki you get Reiki.

Reiki always works, but the recipient may not be ready to release and heal at this time. The Reiki love will stay outside their aura in a bubble of light until they are ready to use it, which could be years in the future. The love from Reiki will never leave them so no treatment is ever time wasted.

In the early years of traditional Reiki, a photo of the recipient was used for distant healing. The picture recorded the energy of the person who was receiving the healing. Native American Indians were well aware of this transfer of their spirit through a photo and this is the reason that, in the early 1900's, they would often not allow their pictures to be taken. In *Reiki Fire*, Frank Petter recounts a story about a man who was trained by a Usui master. When Petter asked the man about distant Reiki, he was told only the wealthy could receive distant Reiki because a photograph was required to receive the healing. In those days the common person could not afford the expense of a photograph.

Extending Reiki to Others

Since those days of old, we have advanced in our spiritual gifts and now have the power to direct healing without the use of props. Our clear intent to help another is sufficient to begin the process. A photo can be a good visual aid but it is not necessary. A physical picture is helpful when Reiki is being sent to a group of people, such as families, coworkers or political and community groups. Place the physical image at a vantage point which will be seen regularly, each time you pass it, direct Reiki to the photo, it is quick and effective.

If you use a photo to direct distant Reiki, it will be continually activated when you empower the paper by drawing all three symbols on the back. If the owner of the photo will place their signature on the back it will then contain their current energetic pattern. When time is of the essence ask for the photo to be sent via email with their signature scanned in as well. That way the process can take place immediately. If none of these things are possible, know your intent overrides any proposed process and the healing will be received.

 **Remember:** Nothing is stronger than your intent to help.

Keep these processes simple; don't agonize over the correct way to apply the information, for Reiki often flows longer than we anticipate.

**Example:** I received a call from a client who asked if I was sending her husband Reiki. I informed her that an hour before I briefly spoke with him. He had mentioned he had a migraine headache so I gave him a practice to perform which I felt would release his pain but I did not consciously send any other Reiki after our conversation. When she returned home, he asked her if she thought I was sending him Reiki as he felt an increase of intense energy for about 20 minutes. It altered him so much that he had to lie down to integrate what he received. Her response to him was, "That sounds like energy from Marnie," hence the reason for her call to me.

After his call, in order to continue to assist him, I did not need to stop what I was doing after our conversation and direct Reiki to him, the work was already being activated by the dialogue we had. I gave him information to assist his healing process and his higher self took it from there. The simplicity of Reiki comes from trusting the process and having a clear objective to help others.

Reiki is such a beautiful gift and as you incorporate it into your daily life, you will no doubt feel gratitude for the opportunity to share this light with the planet

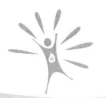

and its inhabitants. Your own techniques will unfold as your practice of Reiki increases. The best way to find what works best for you is to share Reiki with other practitioners. It is fun, enlightening and a wonderful way to honor your gifts and those of others. Check in your area for healing exchanges, Reiki healing or Reiki exchanges. You may find this in a metaphysical newspaper, bookstores or with Google on your computer. The people I have met, and many of them students I have trained, have become my light family and I so treasure them.

 Alternative Methods for Distant Healing

(Using the previous protocol)

The following list will get you started sending Reiki and from there you will find other ways which work just as well.

| |
|---|
| 1.  Obtain a picture of the recipient; draw all three symbols on the back of the photo and write their name or have them sign it.  Place the picture in front of you or between your hands and beam Reiki into it. |
| 2.  If no picture is available, write the recipient's name on a piece of paper along with all three symbols and direct healing to them as you hold the paper between your hands. Have them sign the back if possible. |
| 3.  Make a list of family and friends who are in the need of Reiki and send healing light to everyone on the list. |
| 4.  Hold your hands up and away from your body directing healing to someone miles away. As the healing is beamed to them, their higher self will move the energy to where it is most needed. |
| 5.  Use a teddy bear or doll as a surrogate for a recipient and give the object the Reiki treatment. |
| 6.  Imagine the recipient's body on your thigh, using your right thigh for the front and the left thigh as the back of their body. Do a shortened Reiki |

| |
|---|
| treatment in this manner. |
| 7. See the receiver reduced to the size of your hand and place them between your palms. Gently give them Reiki and proceed to turn them over to do the back of their body. Often the practitioner will sense in their hands exactly where the energy is being received in the recipient's body. |
| 8. Experiment by directing healing to the earth, moon, fairies, angels, ascended masters, guides or your divine self. Often deep loving feelings are returned. |
| 9. When speaking to someone on the phone or over the internet, have a clear intent to assist them and allow the Reiki to flow out as you speak. No other attention necessarily needs to be given for the remainder of the conversation. |

Distant Healing for Multiple Recipients

When I first learned Reiki I wanted to share it with all in my family, but realized that giving each of them even five minutes of Reiki a day would be quite time consuming. I tried different methods until I found one which fit into my daily routine. As I began a self-Reiki treatment I would state out loud the names of each member in my immediate family, cousins and close friends.

I started by speaking their names three times, then I found that even that took too much time, so I reduced it to saying their names once. After a week I found even this practice unnecessary, so I listed their names on a sheet of paper, placed it by my meditation area. As I began my personal treatment, I asked for Reiki to be channeled to them as well. This was simple, quick and I would soon find out how effective.

**Example:** I followed the above plan each day and never gave it another thought. Months later I was conversing with my cousin Pam, who lived miles away. She was one who was on the list. After a brief conversation she inquired

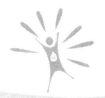

about my Reiki practice. I informed her that she was the recipient of daily Reiki. Pam shared she had been diagnosed with Fibromyalgia three years ago, information I had not been privy to. Her condition had begun to improve at the same time I began sending Reiki to her in this simple process.

So why did Pam improve without her knowing about the healing which was being channeled to her and even I was unaware of her condition?

 **Remember:** Reiki is guided by the higher self of the recipient.

Pam's higher self could sense the healing light coming in and placed it within the appropriate bodies. As the months continued, Pam's condition improved. Pam was opening to self love.

 **Remember**: All healing is self healing.

During the healing process, on some level, often subconscious, the patient has given themselves permission to improve. They allow the medicine, medical procedure or energy to change their vibration and allow their body to balance and heal itself. On the inner level when Pam subconsciously observed the love of Reiki entering her body she opened to it. When she realized months later the love was being directed to her from someone she deeply cared about she let it in even more. This was an opening of her heart and she began to receive love which was always around her.

Don't hesitate to add to your list even those who are not ill, as it will act as preventive medicine. It will keep them healthy on all levels, physically, mentally and emotionally. After all Reiki is pure love, how could it hurt?

When Reiki is sent to multiple people at one time the energy is not depleted, it is actually intensified. Reiki is pure divine love; the more you give the more you get. Fill your list with as many people as you would like: friends, family, business associates, adding especially the ones which you don't have good rapport. Reiki will soften the difficult people and/or relationships. Do not doubt the ability of Reiki. Its divine intelligence will travel to where it is most needed, blessing everyone and everything in its path.

 **Remember:** Make sending healing easy, intend for it to flow into your everyday life and it will be so.

Do not stress about how long it takes to do distant treatments. There is time for all you want to get done. Enjoy it; after all you are just channeling LOVE. In our busy lives, it is sometimes hard to find time for self healing, let alone healing of others, so here are a few quick and easy methods.

 Life Tool: Activating Distant Reiki to Multiple Recipients

| |
|---|
| 1. Place a list of friends, relatives, business associates and others who need love and support beneath a glass bowl of water or a candle. Place your hands over the candle or bowl direct in loving energy and it will be received by all on the list. You may also send the energy into the bowl with just your eyes every time you pass by it. |
| 2. While you are performing a self treatment repeat the names of those who need help or write their names on paper and place the list with their names close to you. Guided by your intent the healing energy will go into you and to all the others on the list. |
| 3. While in a session with a client imagine Reiki going to another who is in need of healing. Reiki is pure love; it draws from the Universe and this love is never ending. It will not be depleted; it flows continuously. |

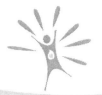

> You are not depriving your client of healing; you are actually adding to it.

Spiral Healing Method

The spiral is a natural flow pattern in our universe. It can be seen in seashells, whirlpools, our inner ears or in the horns of a ram. Even our galaxy moves in a spiral. By mimicking this circular motion, the Reiki healing will be intensified. Create a circle of practitioners in a clockwise direction; they may sit or stand. Each person places their hands on the back of the person in front of them and beams Reiki into their body. In turn, each speaks the name or names of those who require healing assistance. The person furthest from the center directs the combined Reiki to all the people named.

**Example:** I used this method in a class and one of the students had just lost her father. At the end of our treatment she shared that she saw her father in the room with us. He was in a suit, happy and about 20 years old. His young age supported the understanding that once we pass out of our bodies we often return to a younger more vibrant age. This was quite a blessing for her to see her father at peace and it gave confirmation to the class that when we send out healing it is received, even on the other side.

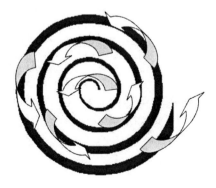

Spiral Healing

Healing intent starts in the center and builds as it flows to the recipients

Life Tool:  Spiral Healing

| |
|---|
| 1. The group will stand forming a spiral as shown in the illustration. |
| 2. In unison, the group draws all three symbols and speaks the names of the symbols as they imagine the recipients in their mind's eye. |
| 3. Have the participants state the name of the person or persons whom they are directing the healing towards. |
| 4. Each practitioner directs Reiki into the back of the practitioner in front of them. |
| 5. The last or outer person directs the energy out to all who are named. |
| 6. Send healing for five to 20 minutes. |
| 7. End the session by drawing all three symbols and chanting the names of those symbols. |
| 8. Turn your hands up and give thanks for all the Great Ones who have assisted as the recipients are released. |

Blessing Bowl Healing Method

   This process is similar to spiral group healing, with the exception that the person or persons in need of Reiki are placed in the center of a circle. The recipients are imagined in the circle by putting their photos in the center or by merely speaking their names. The intent for assisting others will create the connection needed for healing.

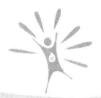

Whole groups may be placed in the Blessing Bowl, such as all abused children, the animal kingdom, a country or city, all healers and even Mother Earth. Each time the imaginary Blessing Bowl is created it can be a different form as listed below.

Blessing Bowl

Healing love is sent to the recipients in the center, then it expands back to the senders.

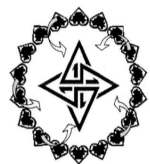

 Life Tool: Imaginary Blessing Bowls

| | |
|---|---|
| 1. | Imagine the bowl full of crystals and each person placed within is a sparkle of light. The Divine adds its light as the presence of each person combines and creates a light force with an abundance of healing energy. |
| 2. | The bowl reflects a ship that fills with loved ones to be healed, and sails out into a sea of peace and happiness. |
| 3. | In the Fall, each recipient is a colorful leaf; after healing is transferred, a breeze sweeps them up into the sky where the lightness of the air heals their wounds: physical, mental and emotional. |
| 4. | On the night of a full moon, imagine each recipient sitting on the moon in the center of the room. As the moon rises, guides enter and take each recipient to a place for their personal healing. |
| 5. | In the Spring, pretend fairies and gnomes are in the circle. They dance with each person who is placed into the center for healing. Finally, a group of angels appears and lifts the participants out of their pain, allowing them to become aware of their own inner light. |

Life Tool: Channeling Healing within a Group

| | |
|---|---|
| 1. | Each person in the circle is given time to speak the names of as many people as they desire to be in the Blessing Bowl. |
| 2. | Depending on the spiritual level of the group the symbols are: |
| a. | Said silently, if there are no other Reiki healers in the group. |
| b. | Said audibly if people are Reiki level two students and above. |
| 3. | Everyone raises their hands, directing energy to the center of the circle. |
| 4. | This technique may be used even if there is only one Reiki practitioner in the group. Draw the symbols in your mind's eye and say them silently. |
| 5. | You may direct the group through the process using the visuals written above in the "Life Tool: Imaginary Blessing Bowls." This can be used to create new concepts, for the bowl will act as a catalyst for new ideas to form in meetings. |

## Healing Past Traumas or Situations

When assisting others to heal a past situation, it is helpful to make the client aware of the divine assistance which is just within their reach. Introduce them to their higher self, for it knows the best way to approach any issue. To do this, use a form of guided imagery meditation with the next "Life Tools" listed. It is wise to start by asking the client to visualize their chakras opening. This will help to awaken their intuitive senses. A Reiki treatment will automatically open all of the

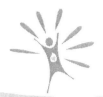

chakras, but when the client is visually guided through the process they become aware of the unseen, in and around them, thus stimulating their creative right brain. They will then be better able to retrieve what is needed for deep healing of their emotional as well as their physical body.

As in the "Life Tool: Releasing Spirit Attachments," direct the client through a clearing of all their chakras and then allow them to become aware of their higher self. Have them step back and view their physical form, then ask to see their divine essence. Start with a sense of color for it is often the simplest to perceive. This is the vibrancy of their own divine light. Next, call in a guide and an angel. The guide will lead them to the original core incident; the angel is there for protection and compassionate support.

Ask the guide to take them to the original incident, to the time frame which is held in their subconscious mind. It is only a story, one the mind recalls, but it may not have happened the way they remember or even at all. The subconscious mind registers information in obscure ways - this is not so much about locating the real truth as it is about releasing the mind from old patterns it holds. Don't be surprised if the first clearing is at a very young age, often we take on issues from our family when we are as young as infants. Use the following dialogue to guide yourself or clients to clear past issues.

 Life Tool:  Self Healing for Issues in the Past

| |
|---|
| 1. Begin transmitting Reiki for about five minutes. |
| 2. Remember there is no need to sense or experience old traumas; you will be the observer of the situation from the wisdom of your adult self and have the assistance of higher level beings. |
| 3. Ask for each chakra to open. |
| 4. Request the presence of a guide and an angel or higher level being. |

| |
|---|
| 5. Bring to mind the earlier issue, emotion or pattern. |
| 6. If the original incident is known, state its time, date and location – otherwise, estimate these factors. |
| 7. Draw Cho-Ku-Rei, Sei-He-Ki and Hon-Sha-Ze-Sho-Nen. |
| 8. Imagine yourself at the age of this situation. |
| 9. Name the circumstance and ask healing to flow to the root cause. |
| 10. By using the mental/emotional symbol, traumatic incidents can be brought into a new light, forming a new perspective. |
| 11. The distant symbol will move the healing through space to the appropriate time. |
| 12. Divine assistance is always at hand. |

## Energy Healing Into the Future

Once again we are reminded that time is an illusion made up in our minds; therefore what is done in present time can affect the past and the future. We create our own reality through the thoughts we repeat in our conscious and sub-conscious mind. Notice how you express yourself both audibly and in silent self talk. Words will immediately begin to physically activate the dialogue which runs in your head, so always attempt to make them positive. If your affirmation is "I am healing now," your body will always be on the mend. Affirm, "I am always in perfect, balanced health." Therefore when using distant Reiki for future events, it is the power of thought, along with the symbols, which creates the manifestation of health.

 **Remember:** Words have power, as do thoughts.

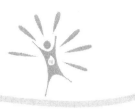

When healing is sent into a future time frame, the energy will remain there and build healing light. It becomes a reservoir of energy so that when you arrive at the time and place designated you will reap the benefits of the process. This works well with business meetings, vacations, family gatherings, surgery and so on. Energy can be sent to a client, business associate or a friend even before they arrive. Then they will be calm and more receptive to the gifts they can receive in this meeting.

As with healing at a distance and into the past, the procedure for healing into the future remains about the same. Naming the approximate date, time and location will direct the energy and expedite the process. If any of these items are unknown, an estimate may be used. Draw the symbols over an appointment book to direct Reiki to clients or business contacts before they come in for an appointment. Reiki can also clear and balance energies for meetings of any kind, family gatherings, personal dates, educational classes, the list is endless. All three symbols are required, Cho-Ku-Rei, to empower the situation, Sei-He-Ki, to enlighten the recipient to new perspectives and Hon-Sha-Ze-Sho-Nen, to allow the healing to move into the appropriate time continuum.

Each time you recall the event, send Reiki to it. When the time arrives there will be plenty of Reiki to draw from, as this process creates a battery full of energy at the location. Once the event arrives the site will be overflowing with the compassion, love and the understanding that Reiki brings from the higher self of each person present. New ideas will be presented, harmony will prevail and all in all, the entire event will be divinely guided.

**Example:** There was a student who tried this approach for a group that she met with regularly. She commented that no one in the group really gets along. After using distant Reiki for the future much to her surprise the meeting not only was harmonious but people were actually laughing and having a good time.

**Remember:** Don't believe anything I say, prove it to yourself by applying the process.

 Life Tool:  Reiki Sent into the Future

| | |
|---|---|
| 1. | Direct the recipient into a place of peace by beginning a hands-on energy treatment which will address the subconscious mind. |
| 2. | In their relaxed state, have the recipient name the future event they would like to empower. |
| 3. | State the date, time and location where the event will be. |
| 4. | Draw all three symbols and state their names silently. |
| 5. | The energy will travel at the speed of thought. |
| 6. | Listen for any guidance coming from the recipient's higher self. |
| 7. | When the thought enters your mind, resend Reiki to the event. |
| 8. | You may apply this process for yourself as well. |

## Memory Storage, the Akashic Records

Energy cannot be destroyed, once created it will always exist, this is a scientific fact. So where does the energy of the memory of our thoughts and experiences go? Because thoughts do not have form we will imagine them as words on a page. These experiences will then be transferred to a place; this is known as the Akashic Records. All of the stories held in our soul are in these chronicles, in the etheric realm. It is a library of the entire life of each and every inhabitant on earth. Within these archives are karmic debts, unresolved vows and contracts.

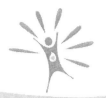

There are times when access to this information can be obtained by using Reiki. Hon-Sha-Ze-Sho-Nen moves Reiki to the place of deepest healing. If that place is in the Akashic records, wisdom will be acquired and the transformation will take place by the information found within these journals.

Begin with the basic protocol to activate distant Reiki. State that you would like entrance to the Akashic records to find information to assist in clearing and understanding an issue. To begin the imagery, you can pretend to see a long room with books on either side. At the door is the Akashic record keeper who is a tall man with a long white beard. Request entrance and see him granting you admission. Continue your story from there.

**Example:** I once used this library to help clients with weight loss. Often the body stores stressful memories as weight on the body. I had my clients put the stories they are holding in their body fat, on a computer disk. I felt this would hold more information than a book and it was lighter, and becoming lighter was the goal. We then shot this disk out like a Frisbee to the Akashic record keeper. He caught it and filed it away. This made the process fun and released the stress of recalling what made the weight stay on; we just got rid of it.

When entering a session, have a focus to make it fun and it will take the tension away from the troubling situation and be amazingly more efficient. It will then be a process the client will want to return to on their own. This empowers them.

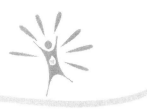

# Chapter 5

## Deepening Chakra Awareness

Chakras are how we interpret what we see through our eyes via the energy systems of our body. The body is composed of more than just physical matter. As you saw in first degree Reiki, there are esoteric bodies as well as physical. The spiritual is about an arm's length outside of the physical body; the mental body is the next closest and the emotional body is only a few inches from the skin. If one doubts the existence of these bodies, recall a time when someone stood too close to you and remember how uncomfortable it felt. It was because they had entered one of your energy bodies without an invitation; they had infringed into your personal space. Most people are not open to seeing this field, yet many people can definitely feel when someone invades this area without permission.

**Example:** Television is not my favorite pastime, though there is one program which I found quite entertaining. There was a TV sitcom in the 90's called "*Seinfeld*" which portrayed 4 people living in New York City and their every day happenings. Most of their scenarios were from real life experiences of the writers and those involved in the various aspects of making the show. This connection to real life is what made the show so amusing

There was an episode where Jerry and his friends were at a party when they encountered a person who did not respect their personal space and would stand very close to them; they called him the "close talker." The next day Jerry and his friends were having a discussion about how uncomfortable it was to be with this man who was very close to their face when he conversed with them. I am sure we have all experienced this at some time in our lives.

The pattern of the show was they would share a strange occurrence and then that character would be introduced to the audience. True to form, the "close talker" visited Jerry at his apartment; watching the interaction of Jerry and the "close talker" made it obvious how uncomfortable a situation like this can be. It is not only felt by the person whose bodies are infringed upon, but also by ones who observe the situation. Because these bodies do exist and can be sensed, it is important to acknowledge them in the healing process.


Body Awareness

These esoteric energy bodies are a real part of our anatomy. To get a sense of them try to open your awareness and pay attention to what you are feeling within your body and then 18 inches outside of it. You will then begin to be able to tune into these unseen yet real forms. Focus and imagine just one of these bodies during meditation when you are alone. Next, be aware of how this body feels when you are with one person and then in a crowd. Notice how each of these four bodies changes depending on physical location and the information presented in a conversation.

**Example:** Become still and sense your mental body, can you feel it in your head or is it merely out in front of you. Now focus on your emotional body,

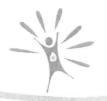

does it sit on your skin, penetrate your body and/or resonate in a chakra, perhaps the solar plexus? As you take a moment to access your spiritual body do you notice it is light in nature, not being as heavy as the other bodies? The next time you are out in public, at work, or with family or friends notice how these bodies change, react and influence your mood.

A few questions to ponder:
   How do we personally access information through our bodies
      and not our minds?
   Can this be helpful in the work place?
   Can we bring more energy into our bodies with a conscious intent?

Sally worked for the Environmental Protection Agency; her job was to make sure companies were in compliance with the local environmental laws. She would visit the sites and determine the level, if any, of contamination. Sally came to me for a treatment because she was finding that employees with negative attitudes were constantly talking to her about their problems. After they left her office she found the conversations would leave her feeling very drained of energy. Sally wanted to know how to stop drawing contradictory people to her and how she could be unaffected by what was said.

My first intuition was to get Sally to feel her own inner power and to learn to honor it, because she was giving her power away during these dialogues. The things we give away first are the parts we do not value within ourselves. Sally had low self-esteem, so she gave herself away by letting people use her. If she could sense the beautiful person she was, she would be able to have stronger boundaries and to express her needs to others in the moment.

I had Sally lie down on the massage table. To help her relax, I placed my hands on her heart and allowed energy from the Universe to flow into her. Then I guided her through the opening of her chakras. Sally then had a sense of her esoteric energies and was able to go deeper into her subconscious and locate new perceptions.

The following "Life Tool: Body Awareness" is to introduce the client to the subtle energies around their body as well as activating their imagination. By pretending to see something, the imagination is primed. This process is similar to how water pumps were started in old farmhouses. Water was poured down the pump into the well and as the handle was moved up and down, the water would begin to flow. By placing water in the pipe before beginning to pump the handle, the pump was primed, which allowed the water to rise. During guided imagery meditations, the mind is given ideas to follow and soon the imagination is primed and begins to create metaphors on its own. Try this exercise on yourself to see how easy the imagination is stimulated.

 Life Tool:  Body Awareness

Use this exercise with one who does not have a full awareness of their feelings, as this will heighten their sensitivity.

| |
|---|
| 1. Sit in a quiet place where you will be undisturbed. |
| 2. Close your eyes and take three deep cleansing breaths. |
|    a. This creates a pattern the body will be able to access in future meditations. |
|    b. The whole body will relax after the third breath. |
| 3. Bring your conscious attention into the breath. |
| 4. What is the temperature of the air in your nostrils? |
|    a. Which nostril is dominant? |
|    b. Is the air warm, cool, dry or moist? |
| 5. *Notice how your lungs rise and fall. Take your time as you observe.* |
|    a. Which lung fills first? |
|    b. How relaxed is your breath? |

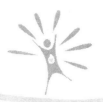

| |
|---|
| c. Let go and just let the air gradually flow into your body and allow your lungs gently drop as you exhale. |
| 6. Imagine the oxygen in the air entering the blood stream. |
|     a. Give the oxygen an image and follow it into an artery. It could be a pink heart, a blue power bubble or your own image. |
|     b. Flow with it as it cycles through your body and back to your heart. |
|     c. Is there a steady flow or does it slow down somewhere along the way? Don't analyze the process just observe it. |
| 7. Follow the toxins as they are released from the body through the blood. |
|     a. If there is dis-ease in the body, imagine more toxins being released on your exhale. |
|     b. All it takes is your conscious intent and the clearing will be granted. |
|     c. You are the master of your body. Affirm any release will be gentle and aligned with your schedule and lifestyle. |
| 8. Move your attention from the inside of your body to the outside at the skin. |
| 9. Keeping your attention on the air, notice how the air feels on the surface of your body. |
|     a. Is it warm or cool? |
|     b. Does the air have weight next to your skin? |
|     c. Do you sense movement, a color or a sensation which you cannot describe? |
| 10. Direct your attention eighteen inches outside of your body. |
|     a. What is the difference between this location and the area closest to your skin? |
|     b. Don't evaluate it; just enjoy feeling the subtle differences or the lack thereof. |
| 11. You are now feeling your energy body, aura or light body. |
| 12. Relax into this new awareness until you feel complete. |

| 13. Begin to become conscious of outside sounds. |
|---|
| a.  Move your fingers or toes. |
| b.  Take a deep breath and open your eyes and feel totally refreshed. |

## The Importance of the Energy Bodies - Chakras

Energy bodies allow one to be aware and to understand the different energies all around. This will come in handy in business, sales, managing employees and getting a point across in business or personal situations. Once you know how your energy body feels while you are alone, you will know if you are aligned when you are in the presence of another. You will be able to understand what is really being expressed without focusing on the words. There is often more nonverbal communication happening than verbal and according to your level of ability to read this information, you will be able to determine your position and next step in any situation.

Know what is behind the words, what are the individuals true desires. This understanding can only be accessed when you have practiced becoming in touch with your esoteric bodies. Then you will know exactly what you are feeling rather than hearing. Words do not always express the truth of another. There is information which lies within the energy centers of the body called chakras and these can be sensed within ourselves as well as within others.

Chakras are anchored in the spine and then radiate outside the physical body into the etheric body where we receive, transmit and process information. They are made up of vortices of energy, each center having a different number of vortices within them. The chakras are about six inches in diameter and can be felt with the hands about one inch above the body. They draw in energy from the universal energy around us, somewhat like a whirlpool or hurricane. Depending on how much energy and information we can absorb at the time, our energy centers will correspond and open to take in the energy. There is so much energy and

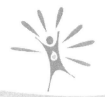

information being transmitted around us that we could not possibly absorb all of it, so our body adapts to the input it can handle by the marginal opening and closing of our chakras. It is quite an amazing process.

If there is a block or misalignment, there will be resistance to the life force running through the body. This will create pain in these energy centers of the body and the pain can be in the form of emotional distress, which I will call a block. This emotional block can create as much discomfort as a headache or backache might, but on a more subtle level. By understanding your chakras, you will come into your power and know your inner strengths. To know your fortitude, you must also look at your inner weaknesses; this will be accomplished by understanding the deeper, more subtle essence of yourself. Reiki supports in the gentle opening to this information.

Let's look at how information is processed in the various energy centers of the body. A chiropractor adjusts the spine so that the life force can run through the body without resistance. When a vertebra is out of alignment, it creates pressure or a block that can result in a headache or backache. An adjustment allows the energy to again flow freely, relieving the pressure and pain. The energy centers of the body are anchored in the core of the body along the spine and have a similar function to the vertebrae. Life force flows through the vertebrae and out into the organs and muscles of the body. Our chakras assist the body in the distribution of energy into our spiritual, mental, emotional, and physical bodies, where we are able to intuit and disseminate the information being presented to us constantly. This intricate body organism moves mind and spirit into one holistic system.

There are seven major chakras in the body but there are minor chakras as well. Every acupressure point is a minor chakra and there are literally thousands of these spots throughout the body. We will address some of these minor chakras in The Five Tibetan Rites. Being aware of these centers will help you in your everyday life because you will be accessing information through the intuitive centers which are in every cell of your body. If we only rely on our eyes and ears for information, we are missing the valuable nonverbal communication.

Let's go deeper into what is processed in these energy centers of the body. They stem from the spine and fan out from the head, forehead, throat, heart, above the navel, at the stomach below the navel in the lower abdomen and in the tailbone.

#7 Crown

#6 Third Eye

#5 Throat

#4 Heart

#3 Solar Plexus

#2 Sacral

#1 Base

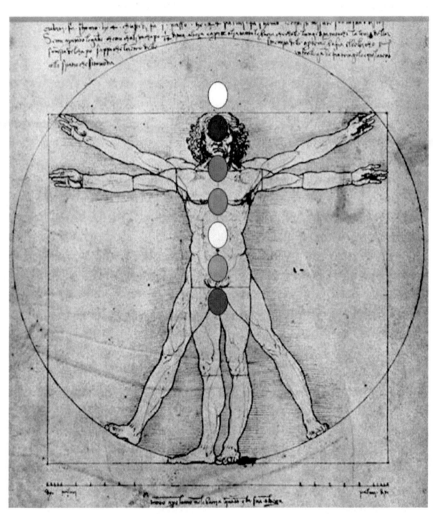

Chakras listed from the lower body to the head

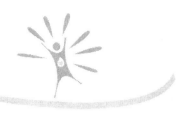

The Seven Major Chakras of the Body

7th **Crown Chakra** Color: white, purple or iridescent light (which is comprised of all colors). It is the connection to Source, valor, ability to trust, faith, inspiration, at one with all life, non-reactive.

6th **Third Eye Chakra** Color: indigo, an intense blue purple. Here is the source of our intuition, concentration, the ability to perceive situations in a new light, choices made for the best of all, service.

5th **Throat Chakra** Color: deep or royal blue. This is where our creation is expressed through the spoken word, expression of thoughts and feelings or lack thereof, addictions, placing dreams into actions.

4th **Heart Chakra** Color: bright green or Kelly green. Holds balance between the upper and lower chakras: activates the yin/yang of the body, love and hatred, giving and receiving, forgiveness and compassion. Secondary energy connects to the chakras in the hands and feet.

3rd **Solar Plexus Chakra** Color: bright or golden yellow. The foundation of emotions seat in this center, rational thought process, full body knowing (gut feelings), self-confidence, sensitivity to criticism and self respect.

2nd **Sacral Chakra** Color: orange. Our creative base, control of personality functions, giving and receiving, power and control, ethics and honor in relationship, blame and guilt, sexual passion and love.

1st **Base Chakra** Color: red. As the anchor to the earth, it dispenses grounding, holds basic needs of life, such as food, shelter, finances, sex, being loved and stores basic family programming.

### 7<sup>th</sup> Crown Chakra

The White energy center is located at the very top of the head. This location holds the essence of spiritual perfection. From here comes the ability to trust life, which includes values, ethics, courage, wisdom and purpose. It is a place of integration, which holds an inner awareness and the connection to all life. This transpires through a pure web of light which fills the earth and the cosmos.

*Example:* It takes courage to trust the existence of a greater plan to our life than what we can perceive in the outer workings of our mind, especially when there is no visible proof. Entering into the quiet of the mind at the top of the head and opening to the universal flow can access this courage. This connection need not have a picture or even a feeling; it is the sense of knowing and trusting that it is there. There is nothing to reconnect to because the connections were never lost. This is the Zen of being.

**Exercise:** When making decisions, try placing your energy on the top of your head, not in your head. This will affiliate you with the courage to carry out the decision received from your highest essence. Now enter your heart and notice if this decision is supported by your self love and if it feels right.

### 6<sup>th</sup> Third Eye Chakra

The Indigo energy center located in the forehead is a vibrant blue purple. In this center, focus is on concentration, self-evaluation and openness to the ideas of others. From here we project our will. We have

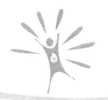

an ability to learn from our experiences, activate inspired intuition, insight, perception, imagination, peace of mind and manifestation.

*Example:* In the indigo center, you can intuit nonverbal communication from others, which makes decisions on how to proceed easier. Valuable information and perception can be accessed in this center.

*Exercise:* When confronted with a difficult person, personally or in business, when it appears they do not understand the positions of you and others, take a moment and connect with their third eye. Concentrate with the intent of entering their thought process and you will perceive how they think and analyze information presented to them. In this space, you will be able to truly acknowledge their way of thinking, converse on their level and find an amiable solution.

## 5th *Throat Chakra*

The Blue chakra holds creation through the spoken word, expression of thoughts and feelings or lack thereof, addictions, and placing dreams into action. The Blue energy center is located in the throat. It reflects how we communicate our ideas, creativity, and it holds the power to support us in following our dreams. In order for a vision to manifest, it must be activated by the spoken or written word. Without verbal action, desires stay in the mind and never come to fruition.

Here seats our foundation for integrity, truth and freedom, which reflects independence, strength of our will and addictions. Yes, addictions; many obsessive habits flow down the throat: drugs, alcohol, smoke, food, even compulsive words that come out in anger and criticism. Creation stems from this center in our capacity to make decisions and in our ability to speak the truth. How many times do not express your truth by saying yes when you mean no, or vice-versa?

*Example:* This center reacts when we are not speaking our truth, and it will shut down in the form of laryngitis and sore throats. This includes speaking your truth to someone else, as well as to yourself. When truth is denied and stuffed away, the body will respond by minimizing energy to this center. Feeling a lump in your throat while viewing an emotional situation is also a reflection of this center. A business guide from the 1980s, *Dress for Success*, told entrepreneurs to wear blue to appear powerful, which is the same color as this power center.

*Exercise:* Try to make a decision or put an idea into action without your word; it *cannot* be done. Actions come in the form of the spoken or written word, which all comes from this energy center. Move your awareness into this center to make your dreams a reality.

## 4th *Heart Chakra*

The Green energy center is located in the center of the chest, it is a balancing center which is more connected to the divine aspects of your nature while the three lower centers are more associated with the earth. This balance holds a yin/yang flow, the paradox of love and hate, self-centeredness and compassion. Forgiveness, peace, harmony, healing and understanding are also here. There are secondary energy centers in the hands and feet that are fed from the heart. We use those centers when applying Reiki in the hands on healing capacity.

*Example:* Why do you think we shake hands as a greeting? Because hands are connected to this major energy center within our bodies. We may rub a child's head with our hand to show affection. We embrace each other with our hands and arms when we hug or pat someone on the back for encouragement. We know on an unconscious level that these energy exchanges are activating the heart chakras from the hands. The phrase "green with envy" reflects jealousy held in the 4th energy

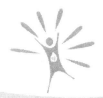

center. When my oldest daughter Carmin was seventeen, she had broken up with her first love. She came into the kitchen, put her hand over her heart and said, "It hurts right here." I could have taken her to the doctor, but I knew he would find nothing physically wrong with her; it was emotional pain she was feeling in her esoteric heart.

*Exercise:* Allow energy flowing from the Universe to enter the top of your head and into your heart. Imagine a color and temperature as you become aware of any sensations. Now simultaneously bring up the love of Mother Earth through your feet, meeting the Universal light. Is there a difference between them? Notice the blending of these energies as they move out through your hands.

### 3<sup>rd</sup>  Solar Plexus Chakra

The Yellow energy center is located one and a half inches above the navel. This center houses your emotions, it is where inner strength and personal power lie, holding your will, social identity, authority, peace, radiance, joy, inner harmony, self-esteem, self-confidence, self-respect and responsibility for making decisions.

*Example:* The unexplained sensations in your stomach such as butterflies, your stomach flipping when scared and nausea when seeing a gory incident are activations from this energy center. The slang "yellow belly" is a term used for a person who is timid and gives reference to the color of this energy center. Intuition is sensed as a gut feeling within the inner knowing in this center.

*Exercise:* Rather than ignoring an emotion or pushing it back, next time, move into this center and sit with the emotion. You may simply be present with the emotion or you can begin a dialogue by asking the emotion what it wants to tell you. To stimulate intuitive conversation pretend to get an answer, continue conversing with this voice like it is an old friend and eventually information will come to mind which you did not consciously make up. Surprisingly enough, this will dissipate the charge or stressful emotion.

## 2$^{nd}$  Sacral Chakra

The Orange energy center is located one and a half inches below the navel. Creativity stems from this center as well as power and control.

*Example:*  Women have the ability to create physical life from their ovaries located in this energy center. As women mature and their life cycle begins to change, they often begin to express their creativity outside of the body. Grandma Moses began painting in her sixties. Georgia O'Keefe was doing extraordinary work in her sixties and seventies. When you are looking for a creative idea, don't look in your head; look in the second energy center of your body. Still your mind and direct your energy into this lower part of your body.

*Exercise:*  Honor yourself as a woman, or if you are a man, honor your feminine side and your female friends and clients, by familiarizing them with the power which lies in this center. Men and women create from this center by their combined ability to create a living being. Women's ability to produce life changes when they enter menopause and this force is then channeled into many different creative processes. They may find that they are now able to bring life into writing, speaking and art in all media. Activate this center by sitting in its orange light and calling in your creative talents. Notice what comes to mind and how you receive the message: visually, audibly, or kinesthetically. Then place it in the throat chakra for activation.

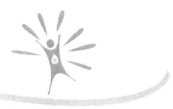

## 1<sup>st</sup>   *Base Chakra*

The red energy center is located at the base of the tailbone. It houses the physical desires of the earth, basic family programming, formulating of the unconscious, passion, power and courage to achieve goals and the stability to bring it all together.

*Example:* When a trauma occurs such as divorce, death or financial difficulties, this center is shaken. It is similar to a building where bricks have been removed from the foundation. The structure becomes unstable and shaky. To stabilize the body and emotions, rebuild from this center.

*Exercise:* When a desire arises for something from the earth, such as money or a relationship, do not try to find it out in the cosmos. These things are of the earth. Connect to the earth and allow Mother Earth to supply you with your desires as it enters first into this energy center. As this center opens imagine the flow as a physical sensation, perhaps a breeze.

For more detailed information about these energy centers of the body, I suggest *New Chakra Healing* by Cindi Dale and *Wheels of Life* by Anodea Judith. These books go into depth about how to work with and understand this part of your energetic anatomy. The "Life Tools" and other guided imagery meditations are another way to access information which lies hidden in these centers. Once directed you will find an easy way to feel these centers because verbal guidance and visualizations will easily open the chakras and release constructive information.[1]

---

[1] See Programs by Marnie Vincolisi for CD's and MP 3's

With guidance through her chakras, Sally had a sense of her chakras and with each session we were able to go deeper into her esoteric bodies, giving her newfound awareness. After listening to negative conversations with friends, co-workers and relatives, Sally realized she did not always help them solve their problems, yet somehow they felt better after they had talked to her. Unfortunately, Sally had become a dumping ground where others released their frustrations and left her drained of energy.

Because everything is comprised of energy, especially our words, thoughts and actions, Sally needed to learn how to redirect the energy of the dialogue she was hearing. There is nothing wrong with listening and supporting individuals when they are confused about a situation. In fact, the process of speaking your problems aloud often allows you to hear it differently than when it is only silent commentary running in your head. I find, as others may, that things are figured out just by verbally speaking and hearing yourself say the words. Sally needed to be introduced to a way of listening to others in an energetically safe space.

There is a neutral space in the heart where one can hear what is being said, yet be unaffected by the content. It works best when the heart center is filled with love. When working with heart energy, make sure you do not give from this reserve in your heart. Always make sure your heart is full to overflowing with compassion and love and from that plethora others may partake. In this way, there is always a reserve left for you and you will not be drained of energy. This is not a selfish act; it is merely wise.

This act of taking care of you first is a common practice. On airplanes, we are instructed to put on our own oxygen mask before assisting others, because we are of no use to another person if we become incapacitated. The same goes for the heart. Give love to others from the overflow of love you have placed into your heart; this way you are never drained of your own heart's love. People who require help will receive your assistance while you hold, and are solid, in your personal space.

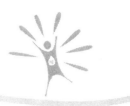

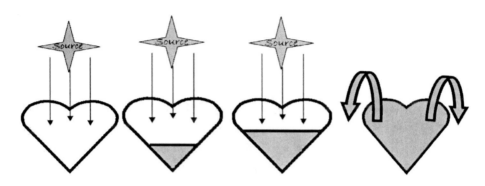

Keep your heart full and share your
heart's love from that which overflows

**Example:** Sally felt it was her job to take care of others, especially family members, because she felt that if she did not help, no one else would. She was taking on more responsibility than she could handle and it was not serving her. I asked Sally to close her eyes and imagine love pouring into her from above, allowing the love to fill her heart. When Sally felt her heart full of love, I had her expand love into the energy bodies around her, the spiritual, mental and emotional. From the space of overflow, there was plenty of love to give out to others without draining her personal energy. I had Sally try this while thinking of her family's problems and she immediately felt the difference, she sensed a lightness in her being yet she could feel she was still helping them.

Sally shared with me that she has a mild case of Multiple Sclerosis. MS is often connected with toxins in the body; it is an autoimmune disease where the body is attacking itself. I remembered that Sally had shared at the beginning of the session that she worked for the Environmental Protection Agency. My intuitive observation was Sally was extending her caretaking role of friends and family to Mother Earth. I asked her how she felt when she saw how companies were polluting the earth. She said it made her very sad.

I saw Sally working to keep the environment clean (toxins) and safe (responsibility) for others to inhabit. The light dawned and Sally saw the correlation between the toxins in her body and the pollution she was monitoring in the earth. She saw how she could release these toxins into a neutral place within mutual understanding space which she learned to use in a previous session. This is where she now will place the negative environmental issues she sees everyday as well as the tension her coworkers attempt to throw her way. Sally now can make new choices.

Sally understood the importance of her job and how she was unconsciously trying to help the problems she encountered by running the toxic waste through her own body as well the emotional problems of her coworkers. This is a pattern and Sally will need to be conscious each time she steps into a factory confrontational situation. She can do it the old way, by running the contamination through her body, or she can allow the love from her heart to overflow and fill the space.

We always have choices and there is more than one correct way of performing any act. The key is to be as kind to ourselves as we are to others. There will be times we forget to use our new knowledge. Give yourself permission to make mistakes and just do it right as often as you can. Life gives us plenty of opportunities to practice.

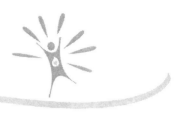

# Chapter 6

## Advanced Second Degree Techniques

Second degree Reiki is not only about learning to draw and apply new symbols. It also includes heightened awareness. The techniques in this chapter honor and help to support these new gifts. To move forward in any practice, unbalanced patterns and unhealthy connections must be understood and then discharged. Releasing cords is one such practice, and it is easy to master.

Divination tools can build intuitive skills and assist in accessing information for yourself and your client. The pendulum can prove to be a valuable tool when used properly. You will find the pendulum chart is a simple way to connect to clear guidance.

As the mind advances the body needs to keep in step. The holistic approach to health also includes a strong physical body which would require daily attention in the form of a simple exercise plan. If the body is not taken care of the mind will deteriorate along with it. The Five Tibetan Rites listed in this chapter will not only help keep the body limber but young looking as well. It activates centers in the body which slow down as we age but this process will keep them at a youthful velocity.

## What are Cords?

Cords are unhealthy attachments to people who have been strong but unbalanced influences in our lives. One is aware of these noxious bonds when there are incidents when they sense a loss of control while in the presence of another. When encountered with them one can become easily agitated and it can be difficult to get back on track. Business opportunities may fall away, relationships could be compromised and there is a feeling of generally not being in sync. This can come from energy attachments which cord or tie us to another person or group, thus creating a co-dependent damaging relationship.

In these situations, it may feel like someone else is in control. But this is not completely true, for we are always creating our own reality. What is happening to us has been designed or drawn to us by our own actions and ideas. The tie can happen when we give our power away because of low self esteem and when we are harboring resentment, anger and judgment towards another. When the connections to these individuals are removed one can quickly feel relieved and like themselves again.

**Example:** As a baby and young child we are connected to our mothers via a cord. One might see it as an etheric umbilical cord which stays connected for the protection of a child during their formative years. This tie keeps the mother aware of impending dangers. This is the line of force which can be understood as "mother's intuition." This is the only constructive connection

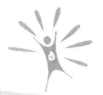

via cords, but this too requires a release at some point. By the age of 18, the cord has served its purpose and needs to be let go. The saying "tied to her apron strings" echoes this detrimental process of being corded to a parent, past the time required. So when a parent can cause a negative reaction in you, it might be because this cord it still attached.

Another fact is that no one can cord you unless you allow it to happen. Even though the attachment is unwanted on the conscious level, on the subconscious plane, you are receiving something from this energetic connection. Your energy or your power cannot be stolen from you; the reality is you are giving it away to another. Once the reason for the unbalanced attachment is discovered it can be seen in a new perspective and easily let go.

The cutting of cords is a powerful practice that can be used in releasing co-dependent energies from business associates, family members, lovers (old or current) or friends. A cord is created to feed each individual in a particular way. These cords are like two-way streets. The energy flows in both directions and each person is drawing something from the others' chakras.

Once the cord is cut, it is sent up to the divine self of the individuals so they may receive a higher level of energy into this once compromised chakra. The release is usually felt immediately. My clients will often notice their body feels lighter and thoughts become clearer when they let go of a cord. This release is permanent because it is done with the use of Reiki, which is love. There is no anger towards the attached form or blame of self during the process. Using Reiki along with the "Life Tool: Dissolving Cords" is gentle, kind and permanent.

Dissolving Cords

How to Lovingly Release Unhealthy Connections

When there is a cord connecting to another individual it will not serve the greatest needs of either individual. When thinking about or seeing this person, you may feel angry, sad, agitated or drained of energy. In a way, they are pushing your buttons when you encounter or even think about them. This can be caused by an energy tie uniting your chakras. Even if this person has passed on or is no longer a daily part of your life, the coupling remains, creating an energetic co-dependent relationship. It maintains its hook through your negative emotions toward them, which holds stress. Understanding what gives this bond its glue, will assist in the release.

 **Remember:** No cord is a healthy cord.

Even in a balanced co-creative relationship, no cords should be established. There is a tie through the heart, but in a healthy relationship it is not considered a cord.

When attached to another person, one needs to claim their part in the scenario. If someone has a hold on you, then you have allowed it to happen for a reason which you feel, perhaps subconsciously, is necessary. Locate the misunderstanding and movement will begin to occur. Holding on to the old story strengthens the link. Try quieting the mind to find the inner reason for the continued etheric union. There is no need to make this a lifelong process. It only takes a few moments to access the underlying information which will release the fastening. The magic appears as the cord dissolves when the new perception is attained. Within moments, relief from the break will be felt.

To discover how one is connected to another, become still and tune into your feelings as you release any thoughts and just be aware of sensations in your body. Analyzing the process will diminish and slow down the effects. Spend some time remembering how the other person elicits adverse feelings within you. Ask to move to the original incident when the tie occurred and observe what age comes to mind. Now sense where you feel the connection in your body: which chakra is compromised?

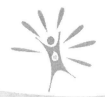

As you feel your body's response, follow the energy back to the sender. What part of their body is sending out a force; from which chakra? When it is difficult to find the connecting chakras, just think of a number from one to seven, the first number to come to mind will be the chakra. This is a way to trick the subconscious mind to release information. When asked quickly the mind will bypass the analytical left brain. Now you have found the origin of the cord and where the energy needs to be released.

Even though it may feel threatening to release the old way of connecting, know that when your chakras are filling with light from Source you will feel calmer. Claim your involvement in this unhealthy coupling. You have been a willing partner in this bond and all cords form two-way streets of energy transfers. You too are receiving something from the tie. Find what you are taking from them and affirm that you will now receive this attribute in a higher vibration, that of Source. Once cut, it is best to send this line up to Source where all chakras should be fed. This will better serve all parties involved.

As you let go of the cord connected to the other person and attach it to Source, you will immediately sense a difference. This process will also help the other person move into a more balanced life, if they choose to do so. Here is where judgment can make a play and hold the cord connected through this adverse concept. We all have free will and we need to allow each individual to make their own decisions.

They may not be ready to let go of the old connection. Give them permission to advance at their own speed. This will keep you from reattaching to their actions because of the opinion you hold about them. Do not let your desire to be free from them, cloud the issues of their free will choice. When you sever the old connection with love it is gone and even though the other party wants the old way of being, it will not happen because there is no longer the glue to hold the cord.

When one finds difficulty releasing another in love because of abuse, ask Archangel Michael to step in and cut the cord. The release will be accomplished with love without needing to actively involve the other party on the conscious or subconscious level. The work is handed off to a higher level being that is all knowing. The client is then free to move on.

Some people are required to be in our lives even though the cord is cut. This could be family members, business associates or former spouses. It is wise to remind your client only the cord is removed not the association.

 **Remember**: Only the pattern is being released, not necessarily the connection to the person.

Once the pattern is stopped it will allow for a healthy connection to the person and then they too are set free. If there is a sense that the person does not want to sever the cord, talk to their higher self and inform them that you are accessing a new way of being with them, one that honors your differences and respects each other's freedom. Even though their human personality may not desire this new way of being because of old patterning, their higher self will always want to improve and clear emotional entanglements.

Unresolved feelings are permanently cleared in the subconscious mind. This part of the mind can be accessed through hypnosis, which is actually a very deep state of relaxation. Reiki as well will naturally take one into this deeper state of consciousness where change is permanently made. Reiki along with the guided meditations of the "Life Tools," will assure permanent closure to unhealthy connections.

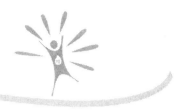

 **Remember:** The subconscious mind rules the conscious mind. When change happens in the subconscious mind, the conscious mind will follow suit.

With practice, one can become extremely relaxed by doing self-hypnosis during deep meditation. Just reading the "Life Tools" will create this state, but for your convenience they are recorded and available online to assist you in creating this deepened state of awareness where permanent change occurs.[2] Once this state is attained, the process will take effect and be cleared once and for all.

## The Process of Releasing Cords

This process is fairly simple and quickly releases those involved. After using the process only a few times, it will become embossed in your consciousness and you will no longer need to read the script, though it is fine if you do. This can be efficiently done as a self treatment as well as a procedure for your clients. And even when working with clients the process can be read, though you will find your intuition will take over and you will be adlibbing and omitting parts of the script, as the clients' higher self guides you to "their" next step.

Start by opening a channel to the compassion of Reiki love for yourself and your client. Direct the client to visualize an infinity symbol of pulsing violet light before them. They will create an image of themselves in the right loop of the infinity symbol and the one to be released is in the left. If this connection has gone on for years, they may see the human images in a younger body. Ask them if this is what they observe to establish their inner sight.

---

[2] See Programs by Marnie Vincolisi for CD's and MP3's

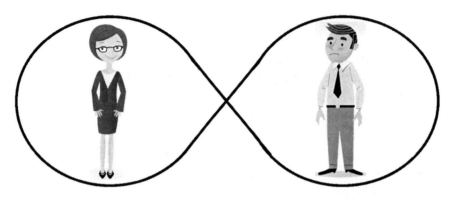

The One to be released    Yourself or the client

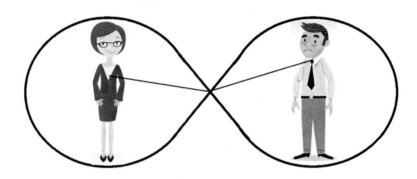

Guide them to recall some negative emotions which are felt when they think of this person or when they are in their presence. To establish which chakra is being compromised, ask the client to sense where they feel this person's energy in their body and make note of that chakra. Next, follow the cord to its origin in the chakra of the other person. Give them time to locate this information.

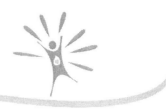

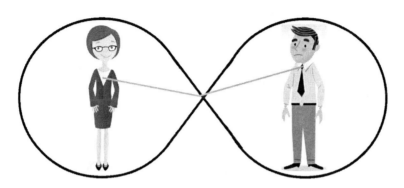

Now here is the key, find out how this connection serves the client. What do they think they are receiving from this tie? When they receive their new perception, often the cord dissolves.

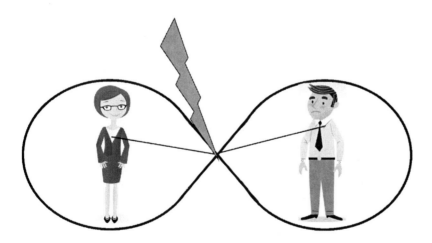

If the cord does not dissolve on its own, it may be severed by a lightning bolt, scissors or by the use of a powerful sword from the divine being Archangel Michael.

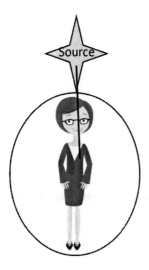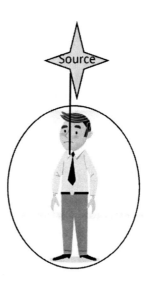

Send the strands up to the higher self of both parties. Once the new higher level connections are established, to soften the release and make the party comfortable, create a bubble around them. Fill it with love from the Universe and Mother Earth. Picture a smile on their face as the love enters their body.

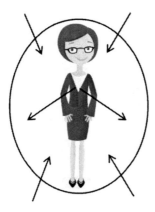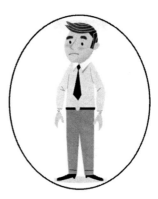

Imagine these loving energies opening their heart, as they respond and relax into the space in the bubble. At that point you are ready to let them go, in love and peace.

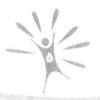

Many times, new perceptions about the old pains are seen as clients move through this process. Let the bubble of the one being released drift off into the sky and see it get smaller and smaller until it totally disappears. Complete the process by filling their personal bubble with Universal love, Mother Earth's love and their own heart's. In the loving space of this bubble, they will feel compassion for the other as they fill with divine love. Have the client accept they have released the old pattern and are cut free from ever connecting to this person in this unhealthy way again. The key to total and complete release is in acceptance that they are, once and for all cut free, in love.

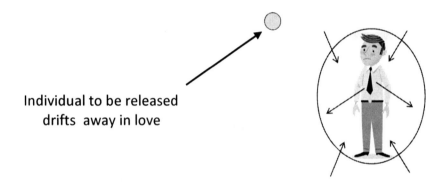

Individual to be released
drifts away in love

Accept you are cut free from the unhealthy connection

This process cuts the unhealthy connection, not necessarily the physical contact. Therefore, if necessary, contact may still be established. This understanding is helpful with close family members and people who are seen on a regular basis. Acknowledge the bond is released as is the old pattern so it will not re-form. This is a very important step, without it they might recreate the old situation. Complete the process with the healing light of Reiki. This treatment is as effective as a self treatment as it is for a service to others. The following "Life Tool: Dissolving Cords" holds dialogue when working with a client.

Life Tool:  Dissolving Cords

| | |
|---|---|
| 1. Slow down your breathing as you take three deep cleansing breaths. | 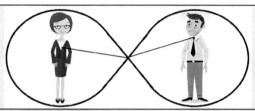 |
| 2. Connect to the channel of Reiki and allow it to flow in. | |
| 3. Take an inventory of your body, observe where you are holding tension and then have the intent to let it go. | |
| 4. Unwind from your head to your toes as you move deeper and deeper into relaxation. | |
| 5. Imagine an infinity symbol before you. | |
| 6. See the image as a pulsing violet light. | 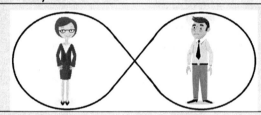 |
| 7. Visualize yourself in the right loop. | |
| 8. The one that you wish to release is in the left loop.          One to be released      Client or yourself | |
| 9. Open to receive information on which chakra connects you to them. Be aware there may be more than one chakra. | |
| 10. Focus on your negative interactions with this person. Where do you feel these confrontations in your body? (Make a note of which chakra.) | |
| 11. As you feel this connection notice where their energy is coming from, what chakra lights up in them. | |

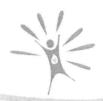

| | |
|---|---|
| 12. Pretend to see a cord connecting the two of you through these two chakras. The cord runs through the cross section of the infinity symbol. This cord is a two way street, it gives and receives energy. (In this image they are corded from his throat chakra to 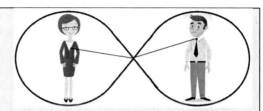 | |
| 13. her heart chakra.) | |
| 14. Before you cut the cord, meditate on what you have received from this person by allowing them to cord into you. | |
| 15. As a new perception is revealed, the cord may dissolve. | |
| 16. Alternative methods to sever cords: 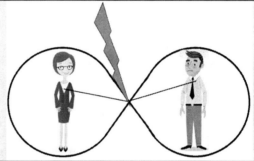 | |
|    a. The cord may be cut by Archangel Michael's sword of blue flame. | |
|    b. Cut the cord with a bolt of lightning from Father Sky. | |
|    c. Connect the cord to a helium balloon which takes the cords up to Source (a nice process for children.) 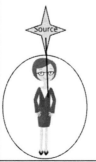 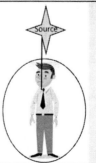 | |
| 17. When the cord is released, it immediately connects to Source. | |
| 18. The infinity symbol now becomes two spheres and each person is | |

| |
|---|
| now in ther own separate bubble. |
| 19. First address the person who is released. |
|     a.  Allow the top of their bubble to be fed with cosmic light. |
|     b.  The bottom simultaneously brings up earth energy. |
|     c.  Imagine the person relaxing into this love with a smile on their face. |
|     d.  See golden light emanating from their heart as the bubble fills with light. 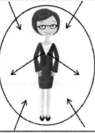 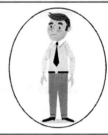 |
|     e.  The bubble begins to move away and floats out into the universe. |
| 20. Place yourself in a bubble of light and follow the procedure above and do not allow your bubble to float away. |
| 21. In the loving space of your bubble, you will feel compassion for the other as you fill with divine love. |
| 22. Acknowledge that you are free and the old pattern will not re-form and accept you are acut free from the unhealthy connection. 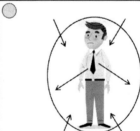 |

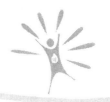

## Pendulums

For every question there is an answer and it lies just below the surface of your subconscious mind. This knowledge can be quickly accessed with the use of a divination tool. The device allows the conscious mind to move out of the way so correct information may be obtained. The reason to use divination tools rather than a psychic is the tools are readily available and one

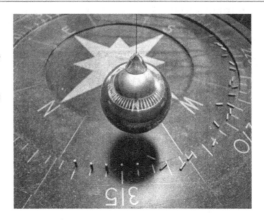

can receive their own truth without the influence of another. Once given the proper steps, it can be very easy to learn how to get clear precise answers.

Pendulums are tools which, when used properly, allow us to receive instruction from our higher self. They form a way to confirm and clarify the intuitive guidance which you already are receiving but perhaps denying. To obtain correct information, open a channel to the higher self of the client or yourself and intend for clear wisdom to filter into your higher self. In this way, the counsel will not become clouded by the desires of either the client or the practitioner.

There are times when the recipient has difficulty accepting that you, as the practitioner, have the ability to intuitively access information for them. Using a physical tool can give solidity to the esoteric advice coming through. Somehow when a client sees the movement of the pendulum, it makes the knowledge you are accessing more real.

When using any divination tool one must have their energies clear to receive correct answers. If you are in a negative space, full of doubt, your answers will be influenced by your mood. The tool is not giving you the answer, the answer comes from within the client and at best their higher self. The tool is only an instrument to assist you in affirming the answers which you might have already been receiving. When answers come in very strong, I always ask to clear my personal opinion. That way I know the response will come from the higher self, not my human intellect.

**Example:** There was a client who was in a relationship which was verbally abusive and controlling. Whenever she asked if she should leave him my first inclination was to say, "Of course!" So before I would use my pendulum, I would always say out loud or silently, "clear my opinions." This allowed my conscious mind to get out of the way and the guidance of my client's higher self to have a clear path into my energy field.

To open a line for intuitive direction, be aware that it is the same process used in channeling Reiki. So it is not a new skill, just one with a new use. In Reiki, we are a channel for the flow of energy from the intelligence of the Universe. During this activity we do not take on any of the client's issues or vice versa. The same holds true for intuitive messages; use the same channel as Reiki and then the information will be allowed to come in clearly and accurately.

Start by opening to your divine source. Allow the knowledge to flow through your head and heart, and into your hands. As it descends into your fingers, it will enter into the energy stream of the pendulum, creating movement, thus guiding the pendulum toward the correct answers. Request the information received to be for the highest and best good for all concerned at that time.

 **Remember:** Time is an element which changes rapidly. The response received is for the time frame during the question. The answer could change the next day.

When the question is presented, the answer obtained will reflect all possibilities in present time. Many questions involve the future and that is when accuracy can be obstructed. Future questions which include the actions of other people can create a wild card. This is especially true in matters of the heart or in

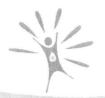

questions about the sale of real estate. The probable new relationship which is seen can change if the other person modifies their direction. A property which appears to be selling in a short period of time could drop away because a new property came on the market which was not there when the question was presented and their perspective buyers went in another direction.

The possibilities of pending love relationships become even more unstable because it involves two different life streams and their free will choice to choose a different path. There are so many variables which play into each scenario it can obstruct the chance for them to meet.

**Example:** A wise psychic explained it this way to me: The vision received could be two people who are seen walking along a street toward each other with the probability they will meet and start a relationship. But the woman sees a pair of shoes in the store window and goes in to try them on. At that point the man passes by and they have to wait for the stars to once again align for them to meet another time.

So when you intuitively see people aligning and then they don't meet, know it is not that you received misinformation. It was that at least one of the people involved made changes which could not be seen at the time of the inquiry.

The way you frame the question will influence the quality of the material received. Pay attention to how you form your questions and make it clear and specific. If you are not retrieving the guidance you are looking for, reframe the question.

**Example:** I will be signaled to change the question when my pendulum swings in a circle rather than back and forth. Sometimes all it takes is to present the inquiry in a slightly different way and answers will begin to open up again.

In essence, we do not need the tools of pendulums, cards or stones to receive intuitive advice, for the power lies within us. We are strong spiritual beings with a wealth of knowledge at our disposal and hold the ability to access guidance for others from their highest source. It is self doubt that makes it appear difficult to obtain. Pendulums can be used to help connect to and confirm new information, but you really have these messages within your being now. All you need to do is claim and accept your power to access this data. In the meantime, you may find this tool fun and useful; just be careful that you do not solely rely on "it" and deny your inherent intuition.

Using a Pendulum

Pendulums can be purchased with long and short cords. A three inch string is best used to find answers to questions, as the shorter string will make the pendulum swing faster. When questions are asked in quick succession, the mind does not have time to form an answer, and then higher guidance will not be obscured. During a hands-on healing treatment, the pendulum can be used to reconfirm intuitive information you might be receiving about the client during the treatment. It will come through their higher self, into your consciousness and then stream into the pendulum.

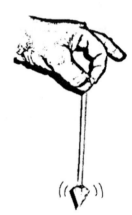

You may also use a pendulum suspended from a six inch string to determine the spin and size of a chakra. Your intuition may tell you that a chakra is closed or blocked. By using a pendulum, you can check the spin and size of that chakra and thereby affirm the original information. If a chakra is blocked or closed, the pendulum will spin counterclockwise or not spin at all. When it is open, it will spin clockwise. The size of the spin will also determine how much light is being transmitted through this energy center; when it swings in a six inch diameter it is a fully opened chakra. Anything smaller requires energetic attention. Ideally when the body is in balance, all seven chakras of the body will have vortices of equal diameter. There is no need to purchase a second pendulum for questions, just shorten the cord of a six inch pendulum by laying the chain over your index finger until the desired length is obtained.

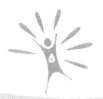

For the sake of practice, hold the pendulum in the right hand, over the index finger of your left hand. The index finger reflects a positive force and should activate a clockwise positive swing. The middle finger casts a negative stimulus and will create a counterclockwise negative movement. The thumb will mirror a neutral charge resulting in no movement whatsoever. Because these three fingers hold positive, negative and neutral action when the pendulum is first being used, it should be held in these three digits simultaneously, thus aiding to the correct answer.

 **Remember:** A positive swing is clockwise (or up and down) and a negative swing is counterclockwise (or back and forth).

Pendulums work in tandem with your intent so you are the one directing the tool to respond in a particular way. You set up how it will swing for positive or negative answers. To teach your pendulum how to respond, think of this training as the way you might teach an animal to follow your directions. Tell it what you want and then demonstrate the action to anchor a clear understanding.

When training the pendulum, present your commands firmly as you tutor. Command vertical and horizontal responses, this is a faster way to receive information. When the pendulum is allowed to give answers through circles, time is lost when it switches to the opposite direction. If one gleans information quickly by throwing out questions rapidly, the conscious mind will not have time to negotiate an answer and then the higher self can be heard. Therefore swinging the pendulum horizontally and vertically will achieve more accurate responses.

**Example:** To train your pendulum swing the pendulum up and down as you simultaneously shake your head up and down while saying, "This is the response I desire for a positive answer." Next, swing the pendulum from side to side while moving your head back and forth. Say out loud, "This is the movement I require for a negative response." Teach the pendulum the way you want the answers to be. If the pendulum responds erratically, talk to it and tell it you want clear answers. It will often respond immediately. For me when my pendulum moves in a circle rather than vertically or horizontally I know I need to reframe the question. It is not the tool which is to blame; it is what I consider, "pilot error."

When checking the energy in the chakras, you may first want to scan the body with your inner eye or hand and get a read on each chakra, then double check your intuition with your pendulum. This is a good way to develop inner sight. Look for balance within the chakras, having them open with equal diameters. Reiki flows through all of the chakras, so it is important for all of them to be fully open. If they are not balanced, perform a chakra balance as described in the Reiki first-degree book, or simply place your hands over the compromised chakra and blaze Reiki into it. In a matter of seconds you will sense its opening by noticing more movement, a pop or just a brief sense of knowing it is okay to move your hands to another chakra.

The pendulum works within three direct fields of energy and they all need to be clear to properly access information. One is your personal energetic field, another is the client's energy field and finally the energy field of the pendulum itself. Even the area in which you stand may require clearing from previously obtained conversations, a sustained auric field of another or discord held in the building or land.

**Example:** In order to get the correct information from your pendulum, you need to make sure all energy fields are unobstructed. To clear the space, imagine a grounding cord on the room, land, or aura of the client or yourself. Allow adverse energy to clear through the cord and neutralize into the earth. Then check with your pendulum and see if other areas are compromised and cleanse them as well.

When asking questions, let go of any opinions about the outcome and do not focus on what the answer should be. Releasing expectation takes practice and you will find it can be quite beneficial when this technique it applied to other areas of your life. When expectations and anticipation are released, so is stress.

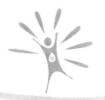

A pendulum made from any substance will work, though wood and glass are the clearest materials to use. I personally do not like wood because I find it a very light substance and does not swing as fast as I would like. Metal and crystals hold their own energy and at first may interfere with correct answers. As you improve your skill any product will work just fine. Remember any material can work when you affirm there is a clear connection to your higher-self. Once you are proficient in working with a pendulum it really does not matter what you use, from a necklace to a button on a string, the answers will not be influenced by the material. This is only a tool; the answers are from the highest source of you and your client.

 **Remember:** Correct responses come from a clear channel to the divine.

To assure the answers received are correct, call in assistance from divine beings. Make sure the help you request is appropriate and up to your standards. Even though they may be angels and guides be sure you are connected to the correct one. Ask for a guide with specific understanding for the topic in question. Otherwise, it is possible to get Cupid when you need Ned the Computer Nerd. Also make sure they are guides whose knowledge and vibration are equal to and hopefully greater than your own. There are many spirits in the outer dimension who would love to play in the arena of earth so be clear in your request. By making this demand you are assured to bring in ones who can assist you on your highest level.

In healings as well as intuitive research, one needs to be anchored to earth for stability and to visualize all possibilities. We are earthbound beings and the questions presented require assistance from beings who possess information held on earth. Events could change depending on what others do within any given scenario. The information you are seeking is coming from the possibilities found on the earth. You are asking to be given what is likely, not what is floating out in the ethers untethered to the earth.

To assure the connection to Source is a clear channel, first perform the following "Life Tool: Preparation for Using Any Divination Tool." This exercise does not have to be repeated each time you use your pendulum. Once this meditation is activated, a pattern is created and your body will remember. Over time there could be an incident which could once again block the flow. When this is felt, a reenactment of this process will clear the lines of flow once again. A cue word will be created and anchored into the subconscious, so when clear communication is required, the recalling of this word will bring the pendulum user back into the same place of clarity as when this exercise was first performed. The word can be anything, a color or an item, it does not matter. It is just a word to recall the feeling of being connected.

 Life Tool:  Preparation Prior for Using Any Divination Tool

| |
|---|
| 1.  Begin by opening each chakra one by one. |
| 2.  Ask to be clear of any programs that will interfere with receiving clear information. |
| 3.  Request assistance from guides and higher-level beings whose wisdom and power is equal to, or greater than your own. |
| 4.  Create a cue word to use from now on to connect to the clearest channel. Each time you use a divination tool, this word will ensure the clearest possible reading at that time. |
| 5.  Visualize open lines of communication from your higher self to the higher self of the one whom you are retrieving information for. |

Occasionally, people may have difficulty getting the pendulum to swing at all. The next "Life Tool: Connecting to the Magnetic Energy of Earth" comes from *The*

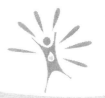

*Pendulum, the Bible, and Your Survival,* by Rev. Hanna Kroeger, an old time herbologist and healer. This method could help with accuracy because it connects to the magnetic energy of the earth. By attuning to the earth's magnetism, the healer becomes an instrument of the paranormal, which are energies beyond the measurable.

 Life Tool:  Connecting to the Magnetic Energy of Earth

| | |
|---|---|
| 1. | Stand with feet apart. Raise your arms so they are parallel to the floor at shoulder height. The left arm points to the north and the right arm to the south. |
| 2. | Hold for about a minute, feeling the magnetic energy of the north and south poles flowing through your body. |
| 3. | With your left hand, start at the right side of the head: Touching your body, brush down in brisk short strokes, past the head, down the right shoulder and arm. Continue down the hip, outside of the right leg and off the foot at the little toe. |
| 4. | With the right hand stroke the left side of your head briskly several strokes at a time, down the shoulder and arm. |
| 5. | At this point cross over the body and use both hands. Brush from the left hip to the right hip and down the outside of the right leg, foot and off the right toe. Still using both hands and short strokes, brush over face, chest and front of both legs. |
| 6. | Recheck the spin of the pendulum by holding the pendulum over your index finger. This is positive energy and should spin clockwise. Now, it should have more velocity. |
| 7. | The middle finger is negative and should swing counterclockwise or back and forth. The thumb is neutral and at this point the pendulum should be still. |

**Remember:** The pendulum is a way of confirming
what you already know.

Do not become dependent on answers from the pendulum.  Know that the answer is already within your consciousness. Trust your intuition and inner knowing. The pendulum is only a way to affirm what you are already aware of.

## Pendulum Chart

Answers received with the pendulum are usually yes or no, but there are no absolutes. The following chart will break down the replies so that you can obtain even clearer understandings. When forming a question, ask for the percent of positive energy and the percent of negative energy towards the inquiry. Ideally a scenario should have 100% positive and 0% negative energies.

A situation may have 100% positive energy, but if there is a large amount of negative energy, then adjustments need to be made before entering into the event. Ask if the negative number can be changed and then intuitively ask how. There are occasions when the negative is difficult to change because there are factors from other people who are involved, which cannot be adjusted at the time. You may suggest to your client to release the desire to move forward in this event until another time when these factors might change. It is likely the desire is being influenced by a force outside of the client's control. If the negative can be changed, then it is likely you are working with the energy of your client alone. By locating the source of the negativity, the situation can be positively influenced or released.

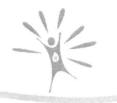

**Example:** Jennifer desires to change her job, but is not sure if this is the correct time. She will ask her pendulum:

"Show me the positive energy in obtaining a new position."
   The answer is 93%

"Show me the negative energy connected with obtaining a new
   Position."    The answer is 22%

"Can this negative energy be changed?"    The answer is yes.

Jennifer will then use Reiki to ask for all blocks to be cleared, from herself, her fears, the new position and any resistance that may be coming from her old job. She will then re-check the negative energy and continue to clear blocks until the negative energy is 0%. Jennifer will continue to use this process as she interviews with new companies, to know where to put her time and energy. She can then make sure there is enough positive energy and a minimal amount of negative energy to proceed with a prospective employer.

It is also wise to ask how much positive energy you need personally for a project to be an amiable pursuit, this is called the personal advantage percentage. Use the following chart to determine this number. The number will usually be somewhere between 85% and 90%. Then, when examining a question, if the positive number is not at or above the personal advantage percentage digit, the project should be let go until a later time. When asking for the positive possibilities in a situation always ask if Reiki or removing blockages can raise their positive number and lower the negative number. 100% positive and 0% negative is the most optimal situation.

To learn more about pendulums and different types, uses and pendulum charts, look at *The Pendulum Bridge to Infinite Knowing* and *Knowing Your Intuitive Mind, Pendulum Charts* by Dale Olsen.  Rev. Hanna Kroeger also has a book on pendulum charts, *Hanna's Workshop*, which ties in nicely with some of her Kroeger herbs. Rev. Kroeger was born in Attabey, Turkey on October 5th 1913 and passed on in Boulder Colorado, May 7th, 1998. She dedicated her life to healing and taught others to do the same. She is greatly missed.

Remember to attain the positive number for the client's personal advantage percentage in any project, which is usually around 85% to 90%. If the positive number received in a question is below their personal advantage percentage, it is not the right fit for that person and they should look elsewhere and not waste their time on the project.

Corrections are necessary when the negative number is high even though the positive number is higher than their personal advantage percentage. There could be interference from another person who will throw off the percentages. Check and see if you have permission to work with and clear the energies of those who are influencing the outcome.

One does not always receive permission to do so. Sometimes it is just a time factor and waiting until another time and doing energy work later may change the outcome. Proficiency with the pendulum comes from continuing to ask questions, I call it tracking. You become like a tracker, looking for a clear path in the wilderness, that wasteland being the subconscious mind of the client. There lie the answers and the place where core clearing will occur.

 Life Tool:  Using the Percentage Chart

| |
|---|
| 1. Ask for the % of positive energy in any given situation. |
| a. Ask if this number can be raised if it is below 100%. |
| b. Present intuitive questions to discover how it may be raised and act upon the information given. |
| 2. Ask for the % of negative energy in any situation. |
| a. If this number is above 10% work on lowering it to 0. |
| b. Bring to mind any adverse situation you may think is interfering with your intent and clear it with Reiki. |
| 3. Obtain you personal advantage percentage of positive energy required to move ahead with any project. |
| a. Hold your pendulum at the base of the chart. |

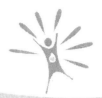

| |
|---|
| b.  Make note of the number it swings towards. |
| c.  It will usually be between 85% and 90%. |
| d. This is your personal advantage percentage. Use it to know if a situation is in aliment with your highest good. |

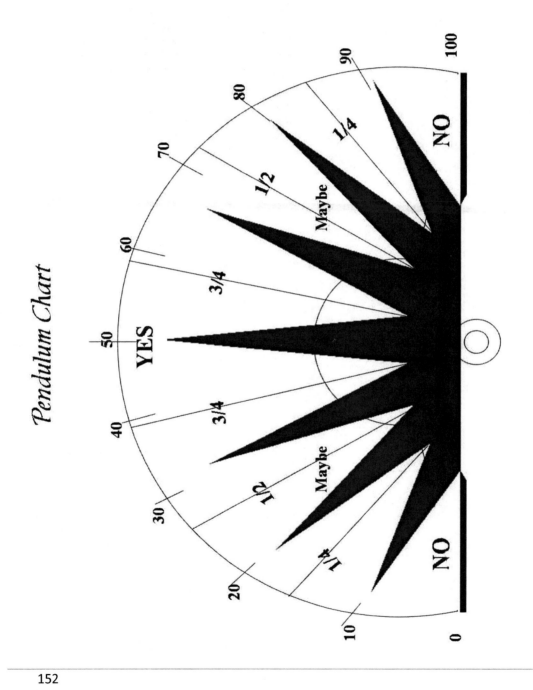

Pendulum Chart

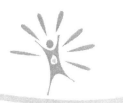

## The Five Tibetan Rites: The History

In the early 1900s, Colonel Bradford of the British army traveled to the Himalayas in search of the "Fountain of Youth." The Colonel had been stationed in India during his foreign service and had witnessed many miracles which tweaked his curiosity. Peter Kelder was an English author who befriended the Colonel. The Colonel wanted to find Shangri-La and asked Kelder to join him in his quest. Kelder felt that an expedition to Tibet to recapture his youth was not something he could pursue at that time, so Bradford took off alone.

While in Tibet, Bradford discovered five exercises which returned a youthful appearance back to his aged body. The exercises were called the Five Tibetan Rites, they stimulate the flow of blood, activate the Kundalini and move the energy from the center of the body out to the extremities. This in turn rejuvenates the body.

The first Rite is spinning in a circle; this activates the vortexes in the body. These centers are not to be confused with the seven major chakras of the body. Their location is noted in Kelders book *The Eye of Revelation,* and I quote; "There are two of these Vortexes in the brain; one at the base of the throat; another in the right side of the body opposite the liver; one in the sexual center; and one in each knee."[3]

The Kundalini is an energy which describes an esoteric fire which originates in the base chakra and lies dormant until stimulated. When it is activated, intense energy will rise through all seven chakras and begin moving the individual into the state of enlightenment. Many Kundalini practices are intrusive and disrupting to the body, but these exercises activate in a gentle, non-invasive way. Performing the Rites will also increase the spin of the chakras to the velocity we achieved in our youth.

---

[3] Peter Kelder, *Eye of Revelation,* 14

Four years after Bradford's quest, Kelder received a letter from the Colonel. He wrote of his return to the states and said he would contact Kelder upon his arrival. Two months later Kelder had a visitor. The man appeared to look like the Colonel, but his apparent age would make him the son of the Colonel. Kelder thought he had come to tell him of the demise of his father, but much to Kelder's astonishment, before him stood his old friend, the Colonel.

The Colonel told the story of his discovery and admittance into a secret monastery. The inhabitants called him the old one, even though many of them were over 100 years old. He joined their practice and had chores to do each day in the fields and meditations in the evenings and early morning. He and the others only slept three hours a night, ate small amounts of food and practiced the Five Tibetan Rites.

One day about four years after the Colonel had entered the monastery, he saw his reflection in a mirror for the first time. He was shocked to see looking back at him a young man. His grey hair was gone, his wrinkles diminished; he was an image of youth. He was instructed by the monks to return to the large city, spread this practice and teach the Five Rites to others, hence the reason for his visit. The Colonel showed Kelder how to perform the Rites and Kelder became fascinated with the process and mentioned it to his friends.

Kelder discovered that youth is found within one self and there is no need to travel to the ends of the earth to find it. Therefore he gathered some interested friends and formed a group called the Himalayan Club. They practiced the Rites and Kelder recorded the teachings in *The Eye of Revelation* which was written in the 1930's. Once out of print, now the Rites have again gained interest as new books about the process have popped up. *Ancient Secret of the Fountain of Youth* is on of the most common books. After studying the original script I see there are a few important omissions in the more recent books.

In my research I found ways to perform the Rites which were not covered in *Ancient Secret of the Fountain of Youth: Book 1*. Those differences are explained in detail in the exercises which follow. The first difference adds a movement to the

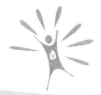

second Rite where the body bends forward at the waist. Another change is in the fourth Rite where you raise your heels in the upward movement rather than dropping them as is done in yoga. Bradford instructed to execute the Rites slowly and to relax the muscles after each Rite, another omission I found in many of the newer books.

The practice consists of five exercises which will eventually be done 21 times in succession. In order to allow the muscles to build and not become sore, begin with only five to eight Rites and increase by one a day until each Rite is executed 21 times. Do not do Rites one to five once and then repeat the series. Perform Rite one five times and then move to Rite two and so on. Once established the practice will only takes minutes a day yet the body will prosper greatly.

*Ancient Secret of the Fountain of Youth, Book 1,* will give the history of Colonel Bradford and an alternate way on how to perform the Five Rites. *Ancient Secret of the Fountain of Youth, Book 2* is the second book and gives a detailed description of the original Five Rites, along with tips on execution, precautions, challenges and easier ways to do the Rites. Also included are Yoga exercises, dietary advice and history. But Yoga is an interpretation which was not in the original writings from Kelder.

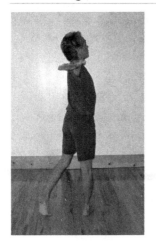
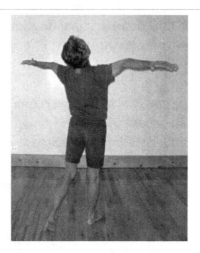

**Rite 1**    Spin clockwise.

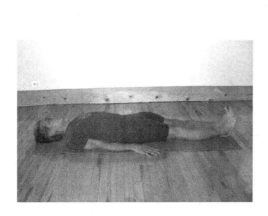
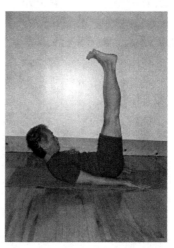

**Rite 2**    Lie flat on floor, raise head and legs.
Slowly lower legs. Relax muscles before repeating.

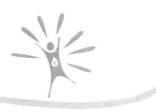

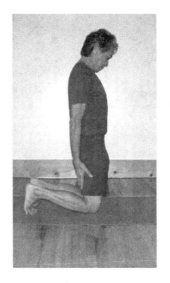
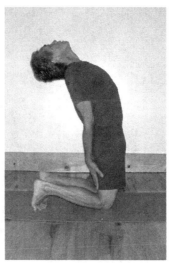

**Rite 3**
Kneel with toes turned under, gently drop
head down while bending at the waist.
Arch back while gently dropping head back.

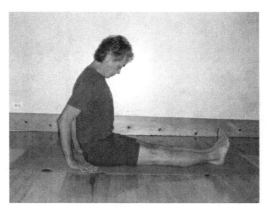

**Rite 4**
Sit on floor, hands by side and head dropped down.

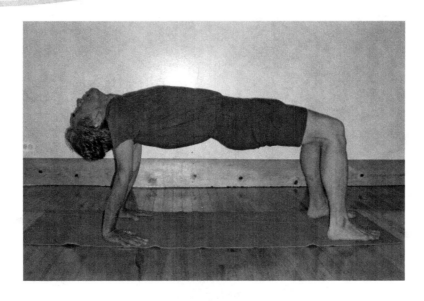

**Rite 4**
Raise body up, hold for a few seconds and tighten all muscles,
then return to first position. Relax muscles before repeating.

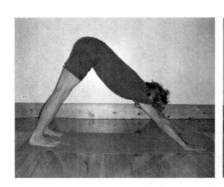 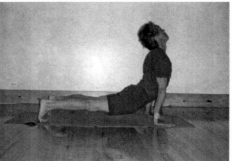

**Rite 5**
Lift body, raise heels and hold for a few seconds.
Lower body, but do not drop legs to floor, arch head back.

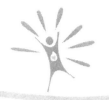

Simplified Process of the Five Tibetan Rites

Slowly build up to 21 repetitions by starting with only five to eight each Rite the first week. Always perform an equal number of each Rite as you increase up to 21 times. I have placed in italics my personal instruction which is not in the original writing in *The Eye of Revelation*. Do the best you can for there are always benefits from performing these Rites no matter what your skill.

Rite # 1

1. Stand with your arms outstretched.
2. *You could have your left palm facing up and right palm facing down. The right palm will align to the earth while the left brings in the light of the cosmos.*
3. Spin around 360 degrees in a clockwise direction. *After the spinning is complete, close your eyes and stand in the yoga "mountain pose" to dispel dizziness.*

*Hints for mountain pose:*

➢ *While standing place your hands down at your side, pull your shoulders back, tilt the hips under. Balance your stance by observing if there is more weight on the front or back of your feet, also observe if you are balanced on the inside and outside of your feet.*

➢ *Notice how good it feels to be a spirit in a body.*

➢ *Once balanced, send energy through your legs and out your fingertips, down into the earth. Sense the energy of the earth flowing up your spine, out the top of your head, pulling your body into an erect stance, as tall as a mountain, yet anchored deep into the earth as the roots of a tree.*

➢ *This will ground the energy and stop any spinning sensation in the inner ear.*

Rite # 2

1. Lie flat on your back with your arms by your side, close to your body, palms flat on the floor. The fingers are facing down and pointing slightly in towards your body.
2. Bring your chin to your chest as you raise your legs to a vertical position, keeping your knees straight and lift your head.
3. Slowly lower your legs and relax your muscles for a moment before repeating the Rite.
4. Kelder instructs, "If possible, let the feet extend back a bit over the body toward the head, but do not let the knees bend. Hold this position for a moment or two and then slowly lower the feet to the floor and for the next several moments allow all of the muscles in the entire body to relax completely. Then perform the Rite all over again."[4]
5. *I found Kelder's above instruction adds intensity to this Rite. It is more difficult to extend the legs closer to the head and when you relax the muscles between each Rite it is more difficult.*

Rite # 3

1. Kneel on the floor with your body upright.
2. Place your hands against your thighs.
3. Turn your toes under your feet (see illustration).
4. Gently relax your chin to your chest.
5. Lean back and arch your spine as you gently move your head backward as far as it will go.
6. Kelder *added an additional movement to this Rite but he gave no pictures for it. This movement is not shown in any of the later books written about the Rites. He says,"...kneel on a rug or mat with hands at sides, palms flat against the side of legs. Then lean forward as far as possible, bending at the waist with head well forward – chin on chest."*[5]

---

[4] Peter Kelder, *Eye of Revelation,* 22
[5] Peter Kelder, *Eye of Revelation,* 25

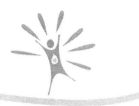

### Rite # 4

1. Sit up on the floor with your legs outstretched in front of you.

2. Feet are hip width apart and palms of your hands are flat on the floor by the outside of your hips.

3. Drop your chin to your chest as you raise your body. Keep your arms straight and your hands and feet in place. Let your head sink back as far as it will go.

4. Bend your knees and raise the trunk of your body to a horizontal table position.

5. Hold your breath for a few seconds and tense all the muscles in your body in this raised position. This will stimulate the vortexes, then relax and lower your body.

### Rite # 5

1. Support your body facing down in a plank position with your arms and legs straight and your entire body a few inches off the floor.

2. With your hands planted on the floor, lift your body at your hips into an inverted V position.

3. Gently move your head back as far as it will go between your shoulders as you raise your heels.

4. Keep your hands and feet in place.

5. Lower your body into a sagging position just above the floor, arch your back, bring your head up as far as possible.

6. Do not allow your legs or knees to touch the floor until you finish the full cycle of repetitions.

7. Tense your body at the highest point and the lowest point.

## Scanning

Scanning the body as a treatment begins will direct you to the body's greatest need. Once these areas are addressed continue with the order of the original hand positions given in Reiki level one, as you continue to attend to the entire body. You will find the second degree attunement heightens sensitivity felt in the hands and increases intuition so that information will be easier to access than in first degree Reiki.

Before starting a treatment, ask your guides to show where to begin, then place your hands in this specific area for healing. Sometimes your hands will automatically move to a specific area of the body as you can just sense where the body is calling for the love of Reiki. Give these areas your first attention as you listen for any other direction from the guides: yours or the client's.

You may also run your hands over the body and notice if there is a slight difference in various areas. The area in need could be warmer or cooler than the rest of the body or have a magnetic pull. Sometimes you may feel tingling in your fingers or in your body when you come close to an area of need. Each situation can be different than previously sensed, stay open to the information you are receiving and become an observer; and by doing so it will increase your intuition.

 Life Tool: Scanning

| 1. Place one or both hands, two to four inches above the client's body and move your hand/hands slowly across the entire body. |
| --- |
| a. Check all areas of the body: sides of face, arms, legs and feet. The back of the body may be scanned when the client turns over later in the treatment. |

| | |
|---|---|
| b. | Need is detected by a sensation in the hands such as coolness, warmth, tingling, pressure, and/or pulling down of your hand in a magnetic fashion. |
| c. | There may be times when there is no unusual feeling in the hands, yet an inner knowing directs you to a certain part of the body. Always allow your inner sense to be the guide. |
| 2. | Trust your intuition; do not think it is just your imagination. Information lies within the subtle voice of the inner mind. |
| 3. | New sensitivity will be awakened with practice. Honor the sensations you are picking up. |
| 4. | You may become aware of the cause of the ailment or emotion. |
| a. | Do not share disturbing information unless the client refers to it themselves as they may not be ready to face the issue. |
| b. | Share constructive information, such as guidance to assist in a physical issue with diet, exercise or the services of another practitioner such as a chiropractor or acupuncturist who may be of assistance. |
| c. | Ask for feedback from client; you may be surprised at what they are sensing as well. This will confirm the intuitive awareness of both of you and enhance the treatment. |
| 5. | After scanning, ask which Reiki Symbol is needed over the affected area. |
| a. | Sei-He-Ki can be used when strong emotions are involved. |
| b. | Hon-Sha-Ze-Sho-Nen is required when the issue is delving into the past. |
| c. | Cho-Ku-Rei is applied when more power is needed. |

## Self Scanning

1.  Same process as above.
2.  Ask for guidance from your higher self as to what created the disorder. *Feelings Buried Alive Never Die* by Karol Truman will be a good reference book for acquiring information on emotional causes.
3.  Accept what is shown without judgment.
    a.  Often we are too critical of ourselves.
    b.  Accept these issues as growth and a chance to raise the vibration of the body and become an enlightened healer.
4.  Be ready to forgive (often yourself) and let love in.

## Headache Remedy

Headaches are very easy to relieve; one only needs to address the area of discomfort with their hands and channel in Reiki. A full treatment is not always necessary, unless the pain persists. First, relax your body by taking a deep breath. Invoke the healing light, focus on the violet color of Reiki and allow it to flow through your head, heart and hands and into the head of the recipient. Sensations can be easily perceived in this high-vibrational part of the body, so pay attention to what you are feeling in your hands as you place them on the client's head.

You might feel the energy building in your hands, imagine this as their pain and pull it away from their head. If you sense a resistance in its release, it could be the client's unwillingness to let go of the pain. This can be felt by the practitioner fairly quickly. Ask the client why they are holding onto the pain and usually without thinking they will tell you.

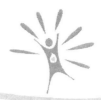

**Example:** I was working on a woman who I sensed was not letting go of her headache, as I questioned her, she said she did not want to transfer the pain to me. I told her I would not hold onto it and the next thing we knew, her headache was gone. When you address their reason for hanging onto the discomfort, the new insight will help them to see a new perspective and will then allow the pain to subside. Often the distress can be lifted away in a relatively short period of time.

 Life Tool: Headache Release

| 1. | Recipient may sit in a chair or stand. |
|---|---|
| 2. | Place one hand on their forehead and one hand on the back of their head at the occipital bone. |
| 3. | Instruct the recipient to relax. |
| | a. Tell them you are not taking on their pain so they may release their pain into your hands. |
| | b. You will direct it away from their body and it will disperse. |
| 4. | Lightly hold your hands in this position and feel the energy building. |
| 5. | Slowly pull your hands away from the client's head. If you feel that the energy is resistant to leave, ask the client to let go of the pain; it does not serve them or use the dialogue of your own guidance. |
| 6. | Repeat this procedure three times. Notice how the energy changes and gets lighter. |
| 7. | If the headache persists ask the recipient: |
| | a. What are they holding onto? |
| | b. How is the pain serving them? |
| | c. Are they ready to let it go? |
| 8. | You will know other questions to ask when you listen to the inner guidance you are hearing in the quiet of your mind. |

| | |
|---|---|
| 9. | Have them focus on releasing the pain, once again. |
| 10. | If the pain still persists, proceed with a full Reiki treatment. |
| 11. | After the pain has subsided place your hands on the client's heart for a few moments and then brush down the aura from head to toe to complete the treatment. |
| 12. | Disconnect the energy between you and them by washing your hands in cold water or merely shaking your hand as if releasing water drops off your hands. Just the intent to release the client's energy also works very well. |

## Hui Yin Position

(hu yinn)        To increase energy while drawing symbols

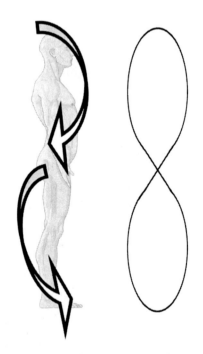

When drawing the Reiki symbols, you may increase their power by activating the Hui Yin. This procedure will supercharge the symbols by bringing intensified energy into your heart and hands. Life force energy flows into the body from the Universe through the crown chakra. It moves in an infinity symbol by passing down the front of the body, crossing to the back at the tailbone, down the back of the legs, across the bottom of the feet, up the front of the legs, crossing once again at the tailbone moving up the back of the spine, to the crown where it repeats its course. This energy stream reflects the flow of the microcosmic orbit.

By placing the tongue at the upper palate of the mouth and contracting the muscles in the base chakra, the energy is held between these areas, thus bringing the full force of chi to the area of the heart, arms and hands. As the symbols are

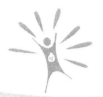

drawn, they will now have increased power. The breath is held while drawing the symbols and then released after the symbols are drawn, along with releasing the muscles in the base chakra and relaxing the tongue.

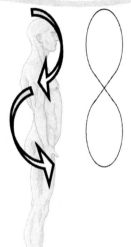

Once this exercise is integrated by the practitioner for a period of time, it may no longer be necessary to hold this position to receive the same effect. As the pattern is repeated, it creates a body memory and it is then fully integrated. The practice can then be followed for personal preference or not for the accelerated energy of the symbols will already be activated. Follow your own guidance as to how often you use this technique. You are your own best guide.

**Example:**  When I first practiced this exercise, I would feel intense pain in my third eye as I held my breath. Once I released my breath, muscles and removed my tongue from the roof of my mouth the pain left. This continued for about a month every time I activated my Hui Yin. After that time my body had integrated the process and I no longer felt the intense pain in my head, yet I felt my symbols were super charged.

Life Tool:  Hui-Yin Process

This shows the microcosmic energy in the body. It's reflected as an infinity symbol as it descends from the head down the front of the body, crosses at the base chakra, and continues around the toes and back up. In this process the Reiki energy used for drawing the symbols is intensified by bringing concentrated energy to the upper part of the body, from the base chakra to the head.

You may increase the power of drawing your Reiki symbols by using this simple process. Once the symbols are complete, release the Hui Yin and continue with the Reiki treatment.

| | |
|---|---|
| 1. Imagine microcosmic energy moving through your body, it enters the top of your head and moves down the front of your body. | 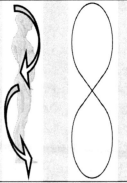 |
| 2. At the base chakra it moves to the back of the body and down the back of the legs. | |
| 3. It moves across the bottom of the feet and then turns and moves up the front of the legs, crossing once again at the base chakra and flows up the back of the spine and across the top of the head. | |
| 4. The stream of energy continues in this circular movement. | |
| 5. While being aware of the microcosmic orbit, touch your tongue to the upper palate of your mouth. | 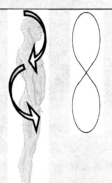 |
| 6. Tighten your muscles at the anus (for men) and the vagina (for women). This concentrates the energy into the upper body and hands. | |

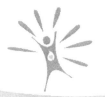

| 7. Hold your breath as you draw your Reiki symbols. You may take a second breath before drawing Hon-Sha-Ze-Sho-Nen if needed. |
| 8. Once all symbols are drawn, release the Hui Yin. |

### Second-Degree Cleanse

After and sometimes before a Reiki attunement, the bodies will go through a change. Reiki attunements raise the vibration so quickly that it can take weeks for the physical, mental, emotional and spiritual bodies to once again become aligned. The usual time period is 21 days.

The first-degree Reiki cleanse often works on integrating the physical body, more than any other. The second-degree attunement generally affects the emotional body but these are generalizations and the experience will be different for each student. The new symbols taught focus on the mental and emotional energies, causing the reaction of those bodies. Self treatments will keep the process gentle and eye opening as new perceptions are perceived.

 **Remember:** Do not fear the process.

If issues arise, trust that you have the ability to look at the situation in a new light and to move beyond the old patterns. As you practice opening to new observations you will be able to hold this focus for your clients as well. Reiki will be the guiding light to illumine old situations and heal through the compassion of love.

The level two attunement will square the energy accessed in first degree Reiki and greatly increase your intuitive levels. With this mental and emotional cleanse, a new cognition will arise with complete understanding of old issues. Often, as you process information about your life, you become better able to assist others to do the same. Stay positive by thinking of this cleanse as a gift which is opening new perceptions, advanced healing abilities and life skills.

### Children Naturally Know Reiki

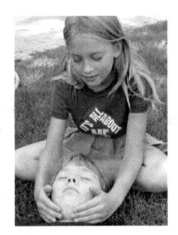

Reiki is inherent within all of us, but children, when given the chance will show how they are quite in tune with their healing attributes. All we need to do is honor the gifts the child possesses and they will expand. Too often our society unknowingly negates and crushes a child's intuitive skills. When a parent or family member encourages the child's intuitive curiosity, those attributes will grow and expand. There is no rule for the age children can be attuned to Reiki. I have taught children as young as six and attuned newborn babies when there is a supporting adult who will guide them.

**Example:** John received his Reiki first degree attunement one summer in my backyard when he was eight years old. One day John was sharing the way he can feel Reiki with his dad. The conversation went something like this:

> Dad: What does Reiki feel like to you?
>
> John: It feels like I'm a brick floating in a cloud.
>
> Dad: Really, a brick floating in a cloud?
>
> John: Yeah, my body feels stiff, but my mind is off dreaming in the sky.

John is lucky to have a dad so in tune with his energy and so supportive of his talents. John's dad, a Reiki master, enjoys gently waking his children by sitting on their bed in the morning and sending them Reiki. He tells me their eyes gently flutter and then open. This is definitely better than a blaring alarm. I am so grateful for Bill, John's dad and the experiences he shares with me how he

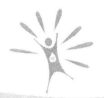

continues to apply Reiki in his everyday life. I am so blessed for the people I meet in my classes, for they continually give me the insight of knowing how to better apply the gift of Reiki, and it is such a joy to observe.

It is children like John and parents like Bill who make me feel very positive about the future of this earth. I do not see our planet being destroyed, for our hope lies within the hearts of our youth and through guidance and love, the grace of our planet will prevail.

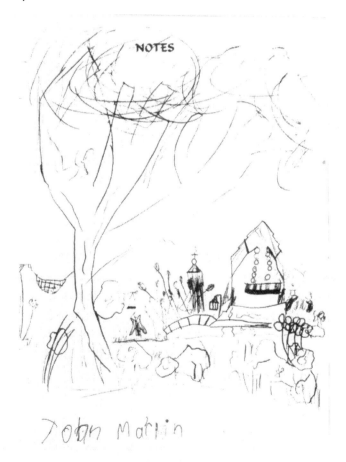

Marnie's backyard by John Marlin, eight years old

"What is a Reiki Treatment?"

This form should be copied and available to share with those who are inquisitive about Reiki or clients who will receive Reiki either in person or at a distance. The forms may be scanned and e-mailed, personally delivered or sent via snail mail. The recipient will then be better informed before the treatment and it will also give them time to form questions. Reiki will serve the recipient even if they do not know anything about the process, but the recovery will be quicker when time has been spent educating the client about how Reiki works. The knowledge they receive will relax them, bring them deeper into the process and give them tools in the future to use on their own. Allow your client to partner along with you and the healing energy. They possess information in their subconscious that will assist in their healing and when they are properly informed, it will more easily surface.

Instruct the individual that Reiki will be flowing for the next three days. It may not be physically present, but it will be reflected in either the mental, emotional or spiritual awareness. Tell them to look for it and to keep a journal for the next few days. The deepest healing will occur when the receiver of the energy opens to their personal healing evolution. If they are not made aware of the changes that may take place, they will go back into being unconscious and will lose some of the benefits of the treatment. Unconsciousness is what started their healing crisis in the first place. The practitioner not only channels energy, but can also play the part of a teacher and guide.

*"Distant Healing Journal"*

These forms are for the personal use of the practitioner to keep track of the results received during and after a treatment with their clients. It is a good way to track how a client is progressing and this will also increase self-confidence for the

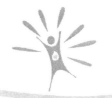

practitioner while supplying testimonials for marketing. Call your friends and family after their treatments and ask what differences they have observed.

**Example:** This form came in handy one day when I was doing distance Reiki for a friend from the Chicago area. I called Michaleen at work just to say hello and found she was home ill. She told me her office had just been painted and the fumes made her quite uncomfortable. She had no energy and was resting at home on her sofa. Naturally I gave her distant Reiki and we concluded the conversation. I told her to let me know how she was feeling later that day. I did not receive a call from her so I initiated the call myself. Her first response was, "I cannot talk now, I have guests arriving tonight and I am cleaning the house." My response was, "So I guess the Reiki worked."

Your friends or family might not let you know how the treatment cleared issues so you just may need to be inquisitive and ask. When people start feeling better they get on with their day and informing you of their progress may not be upper most in their minds. When you share Reiki with other practitioners they usually will keep you abreast of the changes in their body because they are a bit more in tune to their bodies than the average person. This is just another reason to stay in contact with your fellow students in your class and make an effort to locate a Reiki group in your area. In that way you will receive valuable feedback about the treatments you share with them.

"Client Information Form"

This outline supplies an organized way to keep track of clients and their progress. This can be for your personal records or for the state. Some areas may require a signed release before giving treatments; check with your local laws and use the proper forms if others are required.

The most important part of a treatment is the intake interview at the start of each session. If you are observant, the client will tell you within the first five minutes what their problem is, the underlying cause and the best treatment for their ailment. Ask the right questions and your job is easy. Take notes; allow your intuition to open and everything you need to know for the treatment will be revealed to you. Even though Reiki will address the issue without your conscious direction, understanding the underlying concern will aid you in directing the client towards helpful information. This will give their active mind something to think about while Reiki goes in and does its work on the esoteric level.

What to record:

1. The reason for the treatment.
2. What issues arose during the treatment?
3. What were the client's comments after the treatment?

To maintain a client database, use a computer program such as Microsoft Excel and include emails as well as phone numbers and addresses. E-mail addresses can be quickly cut and pasted into an online newsletter to keep your name in front of your patrons.

There are good online services for email marketing which are inexpensive and make your bulletins professional and simple to distribute. Sending out short publications that have information of interest to your readers will be a simple way to market yourself as a healing practitioner. Always remember to ask permission to distribute these newsletters so your publication will not be listed as spam.

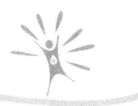

## What is a Reiki Treatment?

1. Reiki works on our four bodies.
   a. Physical: the body and pain.
   b. Mental: thoughts running in the mind.
   c. Emotional: what is felt.
   d. Spiritual: the love held for self and others.

2. Reiki works on the original cause of the dis-ease.
   a. New perceptions are realized as to the cause of discomfort.
   b. Because of the accelerated effect of Reiki, one may feel "off" or unbalanced for a short time, usually not more than 24 hours. This is the process of the bodies clearing.

3. How a treatment is done:
   a. The recipient lies on a table with their shoes removed.
   b. The practitioner lightly touches the body starting at the head and continuing down the body.
   c. The recipient may be asked to turn over to treat places on the back of the body.
   d. Falling asleep is a way a client might choose to get out of the way for a deeper healing to take place. Reiki will still be working.
   e. The recipient will feel very relaxed which will allow them to release their thoughts and receive the full benefit of the treatment.
   f. Treatments can also be performed while the individual is sitting in a chair or at a distance, when the client is unable to be physically present.

4. Reiki will continue to work for three days after the treatment. Therefore, for chronic problems, the best results will be obtained when the sessions are repeated every three or four days for at least three consecutive treatments.

a. The initial treatment will relax the body; after this calmness subsides, the energy will still be felt either mentally, emotionally or spiritually, or any combination of these.

b. A mental clearing stills the mind (allowing one to sleep) or Reiki can bring in a feeling of being unfocused.

c. Emotional release may bring up tears, which are sometimes unexplainable. This can happen when feeling unconditional love.

d. A spiritual healing may awaken a sense for the love of nature, a feeling of gratitude or peaceful thoughts.

e. All of these feelings will subside at the end of three days as new perceptions are realized.

f. Watch how you perceive stressful situations. Are you less attached to the outcome?

g. Notice how you are remembering old negative situations. Do they hold less of a charge?

h. Reiki works 100% of the time. Watch for where the healing is occurring: physically, mentally, emotionally and/or spiritually.

~ *Reiki is pure love* ~

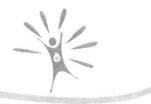

## Client Information Form

I, the undersigned, understand the Reiki session is for the purpose of assisting in stress reduction and relaxation. I understand very clearly a Reiki session is not a substitute for medical or psychological diagnosis and treatment. Reiki practitioners do not diagnose conditions, nor do they prescribe or perform medical treatment, nor prescribe substances, nor interfere with the treatment of a licensed medical professional. It is recommended I see a licensed physician or other licensed health care professional for any physical or psychological ailments I have.

Signature: _____ Date: _____

Print Name: _____

Address: _____

City: _____ State: _____

Zip Code: ____ e-mail: _____

Phone – Home: _____ Work: _____ Cell: _____

| Session Date | Remarks | Progress and Treatment |
|---|---|---|
|  |  |  |
|  |  |  |
|  |  |  |
|  |  |  |
|  |  |  |
|  |  |  |
|  |  |  |
|  |  |  |
|  |  |  |
|  |  |  |

## Progress and Treatment Report

| Date | Clients Remarks | Progress and Treatment |
|------|-----------------|------------------------|
|      |                 |                        |
|      |                 |                        |
|      |                 |                        |
|      |                 |                        |
|      |                 |                        |
|      |                 |                        |
|      |                 |                        |
|      |                 |                        |
|      |                 |                        |
|      |                 |                        |
|      |                 |                        |
|      |                 |                        |
|      |                 |                        |
|      |                 |                        |
|      |                 |                        |
|      |                 |                        |
|      |                 |                        |
|      |                 |                        |
|      |                 |                        |
|      |                 |                        |
|      |                 |                        |

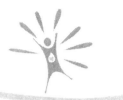

Cleansing Journal

Using the journal will keep the student aware of their rising vibration in each of the four bodies and all seven chakras. It will assist to ground the incoming light and to keep one in the present time. Make the memoranda short to encourage and support the process each day.

Day   1                      Chakra  1

_____
_____
_____
_____
_____
_____
_____

Day   2                      Chakra  2

_____
_____
_____
_____
_____
_____

Day   3                      Chakra  3

_____
_____
_____
_____
_____
_____

Day   4                    Chakra 4

_____
_____
_____
_____
_____
_____

Day   5                    Chakra 5

_____
_____
_____
_____
_____
_____

Day   6                    Chakra 6

_____
_____
_____
_____

Day   7                    Chakra 7

_____
_____
_____
_____
_____
_____
_____

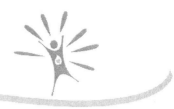

Day  8                    Chakra  1

_____
_____
_____
_____
_____
_____
_____

Day  9                    Chakra  2

_____
_____
_____
_____
_____

Day  10                   Chakra  3

_____
_____
_____
_____
_____
_____

Day  11                   Chakra  4

_____
_____
_____
_____
_____
_____

Day  12                    Chakra  5

_____
_____
_____
_____
_____
_____

Day  13                    Chakra  6

_____
_____
_____
_____
_____
_____

Day  14                    Chakra  7

_____
_____
_____
_____
_____
_____

Day  15                    Chakra  1

_____
_____
_____
_____
_____
_____

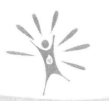

Day 16            Chakra 2

_____

_____

_____

_____

_____

_____

Day 17            Chakra 3

_____

_____

_____

_____

_____

Day 18            Chakra 4

_____

_____

_____

_____

_____

Day 19            Chakra 5

_____

_____

_____

_____

_____

_____

_____

Day  20                   Chakra  6

_____
_____
_____
_____
_____

Day  21                   Chakra  7

_____
_____
_____
_____
_____
_____

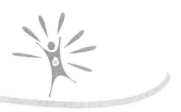

## Afterword

You have now stepped upon the next rung of the ladder of awareness and life changing possibilities. By applying the "Life Tools" found in this book you can clear lifetimes of fear and control. You are no longer a victim of the situations which arise around you. You can now become familiar with your power and use it for your growth and advantage in everyday situations for yourself and those around you. By applying the methods presented in this book, you have no doubt discovered you can make a difference in your world and the world of others, by your conscious thoughts and channeling the love of Reiki.

Now that you have uncovered your inner gift no one can take it away from you or deny that you have it. As you learn how to apply the knowledge tucked away in the pages of this book do not let the processes given diminish your intuitive wisdom. Follow the examples and use them as guidelines only. This will allow you to be open to hear and acknowledge your divine intelligence which is ever present. Once you have attained this light you can move into a space of accepting that anything you desire is at your finger tips. It does not take years of practice to channel gifts for yourself and others. All it takes is the ability to channel love into every situation and all will fall into divine order. Let go of how things should be and the Universe will supply you in ways you have never even dreamed of.

You may receive your second degree Reiki attunement from a local master teacher, from me via the web or ask your divine self to download the energy into your body and consciousness.

As you begin to walk your path of truth others around you will be encouraged to follow your lead. You are not responsible for the actions made by others and what they choose to do. You can now stand merely as an example of the positive possibilities which can be attained when living with an open heart.

I invite you to dance with me on this path of light. We travel along with the many enlightened beings that have gone before us. We are not alone on this journey.

I bless you on your journey my dear divine spirits.

*Marnie Vincolisi*

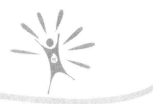

## Appendix

The following books will increase your understanding of how to focus upon and move energy. It is in the practice where the student advances.

*Reiki: a Torch in Daylight* by Karyn Mitchell: good processes with Reiki second degree symbols.

*Hands of Light* by Barbara Ann Brennan: a healer's Bible, packed with information. It can take years to get through the information in this book. Brennan is very left-brain oriented and precise. It is a well-written book including many exercises for tuning into chakras and auras.

*The Pendulum Bridge to Infinite Knowing* and *Pendulum Charts* by Dale Olsen: precise understanding of pendulums and how they work. It contains numerous charts on everything from health to auto repair.

*Hanna's Workshop* by Rev. Hanna Kroeger: pendulum charts and herbal charts to expand the healer in all of us.

*Wheels of Life* by Anodea Judith: in depth information on chakras and chakra exercises.

*The Eye of Revelation* by Peter Kelder: the original manuscript of the *Five Tibetan Rites* with editing by J.W. Watt while the original words of Kelder are left unabridged.

*Ancient Secret of the Fountain of Youth* by Peter Kelder: a fascinating book from the 1930's, which includes exercises to keep the body young.

*Reiki Fire* by Frank Petter: new information on the origin of the Reiki history and Mikao Usui.

## Movies

Movies can very aptly clarify esoteric concepts which often appear to be unexplainable while provoking the thought, "Can what is portrayed on the screen actually be real?" You may reference movies to help yourself or clients attain a deeper understanding for what is being channeled through a healing treatment.

*Contact*, Robert Zemeckis, 1997 starring Jodi Foster, adapted from the novel by Carl Sagan. Jodi Foster plays a scientist who finds strong evidence of extraterrestrial life and our ability to traverse time and space.

*The Da Vinci Codes,* Ron Howard, 2006. If you set aside the religious implications of the movie you can pick up on references made to the power held within the Vesica Pisces and sacred geometry.

*The Matrix*, Larry and Andy Wachowski, 1999. Keanu Reeves plays Neo, a character in the future where reality is perceived by humans as a Matrix. It looks at the reality of the conscious and subconscious mind where people need to be freed from the "dream world" and brought back into reality.

*The Sixth Sense*, M. Night Shyamalan, 1999. Bruce Willis has the audience fooled during most of the movie. It supports the idea of how out of body forms can communicate and interact with those of us in physical bodies. And that those interactions have purpose.

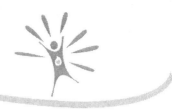

## Bibliography

Abravanel, Elliot. *Dr. Abravanel's Body Type Diet and Lifetime Nutrition Plan.* New York, New York: Bantum Books, 1983.

D'Adamo, Peter. *Eat Right for your Type.* New York, New York: Penguin Putnam, 1996.

Dale, Cyndy. *New Chakra Healing.* St. Paul MI: Llewellyn, 1996.

Grey, Alex. *Sacred Mirrors.* Rochester VT: Inner Traditions International, 1990.

Hay, Louise. *Heal Your Body.* Carson, CA: Hay House, Inc., 1982.

Heller, Richard and Rachael. *The Carbohydrate Addict's Lifespan Program.* New York, New York: Penguin Books, 1993.

Judith, Anodea. *Wheels of Life.* St. Paul MI: Llewellyn, 1999.

Kelder, Peter. *The Eye of Revelation.* Booklocker, 2008.

Kelder, Peter. *Ancient Secret of the Fountain of Youth: Book 1, and Book 2* New York, New York, Doubleday, 1998.

Kroeger, Rev. Hanna. *The Pendulum, the Bible, and Your Survival. Hanna's Workshop.* Boulder CO:

Mitchell, Karyn. *Reiki: A Torch in Daylight.* St. Charles, IL: Mind Rivers Publishing, 1994.

Olsen, Dale. *Knowing Your Intuitive Mind, Pendulum Charts.* Eugene, OR: Crystalline Publications, 1989.

Olsen, Dale. *The Pendulum Bridge to Infinite Knowing* Eugene, OR: Crystalline Publications, 1996.

Petter, Frank Arjava. *Reiki Fire.* Netherlands: Motilal Banarsidass: Publishers Private Limited, 1997.

Truman, Karol. *Feelings Buried Alive Never Die*. St. George, UT: Olympus Distributing, 1991.

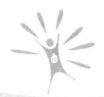

# Index

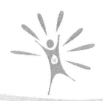

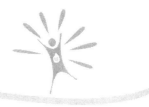

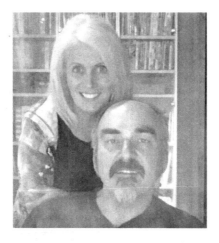

Marnie and her husband Bob

Marnie Vincolisi has been lecturing on Reiki, metaphysics and spiritual growth for decades. Some of the classes she has developed are on subjects as varied as divination, light body work, space clearing, axiatonal alignment, sacred geometry, meditation and ascended masters. Marnie currently lives in Tucson, Arizona and Denver, Colorado, she travels to lecture and gives attunements and treatments to clear and balance the bodies remotely. Her treatments are for optimal health, emotional balance, mental clarity, guidance and spiritual connection.

Marnie's meditation CDs and MP3s may be found at
www.lightinternal.com
You may contact Marnie for personal sessions at
marnie@lightinternal.com

Programs by Marnie Vincolisi

Presentation slides to support the study of Reiki, graphically illustrate the methods presented in this and other books by Marnie Vincolisi. The slides are suitable for class presentations and are available through Light Internal for $39.95.

*Finding Your Inner Gift, the Ultimate Reiki One Manual*
*Inner Gifts Uncovered, Continuing on the Path of Self*
    *Empowerment and Reiki*
*Claiming Your Inner Gifts, Mastering your Life and Reiki*

*Meditation Made Easy* and *Cosmic Connections* feature the melodic voice of Marnie Vincolisi in CD format. The CDs may be used for understanding our chakra systems through guided imagery meditation and for meditations during the attunement process for Reiki Master Teachers. Also found on *Meditation Made Easy* is the process for a Reiki self treatment, easily guided by Marnie, each available for $18.95 or order as an MP3 online at **www.lightinternal.com**

CPSIA information can be obtained at www.ICGtesting.com
Printed in the USA
BVOW030905280313

316540BV00012B/7/P